How to Raise an
Exceptional Child

Almine

Published by Spiritual Journeys LLC

Copyright 2010 MAB 998 Megatrust

By Almine
Spiritual Journeys LLC
P.O. Box 300
Newport, Oregon 97365

Website: www.spiritualjourneys.com
Toll-free number 877 552-5646

Contributors:
Almine Barton, Jr., L.Ac, C.F.T.
Rory C. Mullin, MSc

Cover Layout by Pete McKee

Manufactured in the United States of America

ISBN 978-1-934979-11-2 (Softcover)
ISBN 978-1-934070-73-4 (Adobe Reader)

TABLE OF CONTENTS

ABOUT THE AUTHOR

Almine is called by His Excellency Armen Sarkissian, astro-physicist at Cambridge University, "One of the most remarkable lives of our time."

She is the author of 25 books and founder of the Institute of Applied Mysticism for the study of advanced metaphysical concepts.

This book has been created in response to direct requests from Almine's global audience to provide advice for parents of children of advanced consciousness.

> *"I'm really impressed with Almine and the integrity of her revelations. My respect for her is immense and I hope that others will find as much value in her teachings as I have."*
>
> —*Dr. Fred Bell, Former NASA Scientist*

DISCLAIMER

The views in this book are personal to the author and do nor purport to be medical advice. Consult a naturopathic physician or medical doctor when in doubt.

The author or Spiritual Journeys LLC cannot be held responsible or liable for any practices given in this book as they are the personal experiences of the author in raising children.

INTRODUCTION

They walk among us seemingly as ordinary children. But then we look again, for something in their eyes catches our attention – a certain knowingness, an ancient wisdom coupled with a purity so profound that it stops us in our tracks. Surely the masters throughout the ages, the light-bearers of humanity, looked out at the world with just such clarity.

They may sit in a highchair with egg on their faces but they wear it with dignity, like a monarch wearing a bejeweled crown. They watch us with a benign tolerance that leaves us wondering whether they view themselves as the parents and us as the children.

Whether they shrink from the abrasive and intrusive presence of the world or reach eagerly for it with dimpled, chubby hands, their courage and determination is evident from their very first faltering step. When finally they can speak, their questions are startling in their probing simplicity and their observations spellbinding in their elegant perceptiveness. These are the exceptional children we are privileged to parent.

THE SOCIALLY CONDITIONED PARENT

The socially conditioned parent is locked behind the prison bars of belief systems. The exceptional cannot take wing within conformity. If we have spent our lives bound by the worldviews of others, let us pause and consider whether we wish to subject our children to the same; whether we would ask them to conform to the madness of the world and call it sanity. If not, our child may be our liberation and salvation; the one who will allow us to claim for ourselves as well as them the priceless gift of freedom from societal bondage.

The great fear of parents is that they might make mistakes that could irrevocably damage their children. Driven by self-doubt, they override their parental instincts in favor of outside authority figures. Life supports the raising of the young as evidenced throughout nature. Why would it be any different for human beings? All we have to do is listen to our instincts and our child.

Do not accept that because others vaccinate their children that it is necessarily the right decision. The very fact that autoimmune diseases have increased dramatically since the 1950's should be impetus enough to become properly informed, and then to follow our inner guidance. Inner guidance is invaluable in traversing the pitfalls of life. How can we keep it alive and well in our children if we deny it in ourselves?

All over the world, parents rush for outside assistance for that which can be helped with simple home remedies. Medicine has become big business. Yet 2010 saw cancer overtake cardiovascular disease as the leading cause of death, with an estimated 12 million cancer cases worldwide, 7.6 million of which were estimated to be fatal. Clearly, general health concerns are on the rise.

The health-promoting effects of a peaceful, nurturing home life are incalculable. The self-sovereignty of a child raised to understand and master the symptoms of his or her body, more so. The incentive to raise our children as masters of consciousness can be found everywhere in the ailing world around us. They come bearing gifts of the spirit to be the wayshowers of humanity. All we, their parents, have to do is set them free. Let the journey begin ---

DO'S AND DON'TS FOR A PARENT

The Seven Cardinal "Don'ts"

1. Never give food as a reward. It leads to food binges or cravings in later life when self-esteem is low.

2. Never criticize or reprimand a child in front of others. They become desensitized to avoid the shame.

3. Never over-emphasize accomplishments only when praising your child. Value them for who they are, not just for what they do.

4. Never confuse firmness with anger. The exceptional child needs gentle firmness.

5. Never just say 'No' without explaining why. Dictatorial parents raise rebellious children.

6. Never have marital arguments in front of children or within their hearing. It creates insecurity in them that could affect them all their lives.

7. Never turn a child into a confidant, telling him your troubles or putting him in a position of having to take sides. Allow him his childhood – he can only enjoy it once.

The Seven Cardinal "Dos"

1. Tell your child you love him or her often. Assuming they know is not enough.

2. Silence your mind when your child speaks, that you may fully assimilate the meaning behind the words.

3. Show your child physical affection daily. Loving touch develops nerve synapse function.

4. Trust your parental instincts and your discernment as to when to seek professional assistance. Get second opinions when in doubt. But remember, miracles happen regularly; they are the daily fare of one who has stepped beyond human boundaries.

5. Instill through example the unshakeable faith that life is a grand adventure waiting to reveal its secrets and jewels of perfection.

6. Use your child's missteps as teaching moments. With gentle firmness, withhold benefits to enforce guidance if that is needed. An enlightened relationship has no room for blame – ever.

7. Encourage self-honesty. Indulging another's self-deceit is a great disservice. Praise integrity and moral courage.

> *"To thine own self be true, and it must follow as the night the day, that thou canst not then be false to any man."*
> —William Shakespeare

Symptoms of Disease –
the Language of the Spirit

"Disease and injury can come in an instant – so can healing.

The body is a fluid vehicle of a being as vast as the cosmos, having a human experience."

—Almine

"A truly good physician first finds the cause of the illness. Having found that out, he first tries to cure it by food. Only when food has failed does he prescribe medication."
—Sun Si Mo, 7th Century A.D.

TEACHING YOUR CHILD TO MASTER DISEASE

My daughter was very sickly and abused through neglect when I adopted her at nine months of age. The wisdom gathered here has been born of our experience as Jaylene transitioned into a healthy, happy and flourishing eleven-year-old.

During these eleven years she has never needed the care of a medical physician other than for one foolish trip to the emergency room when she had a bloody nose. The diagnosis given there was, "She has a bloody nose." That cost me several hundred dollars and I have learned since to trust my inner knowingness about what is best for my daughter and when a physician's care might be needed. Thankfully that need has not arisen.

I remain a firm conscientious objector to immunizations as I observe the rampant autoimmune diseases and inflammatory conditions in the now-older generations that were immunized as a matter of course.

Some suggested reading to study the possible hazards of immunizations:
- *A Shot in the Dark*, by Harris L. Coulter and Barbara Loe Fisher
- *The Douglass Report*, by Dr. William Campbell Douglass II, M.D.
- html www.know-vaccines.org/controversy.html
- www.todayschiropractic.com

In raising an exceptional child, one cannot follow mass consensus. When you are training an eagle to fly you must leave the flocks of other birds behind.

Looking at Disease in a Different Way

The symptoms of injuries and disease should be described as the body speaking to us. In understanding the language of pain[1] the parent can ask the right questions to help the child see what area of his or her life needs to be healed.

---

1 See Appendix I, The Language of Pain.

Jaylene was taught that it is not her body that needs healing but her life. In eleven years she has not had aspirin (it is not advisable for anyone not yet 16 years of age as it has been known to cause Reye's Syndrome, which has claimed the lives of many children and teenagers), hardly ever has she had cough medicine or other over-the-counter drugs that so many children are given routinely.

She may experience a common cold every few years. When she does, it is healed within 24 hours in the following way:

Possible Scenario:
Mom: When there's mucous in your head it means you are seeing or hearing low, undesirable messages. What is this trying to tell you?
J.: When I wait to be picked up from school, an older boy using the f-word a lot comes and tells me dirty jokes.
Mom: Is there any other reason you are trying to get sick?
J.: I'm so bored at school. It's the same old thing every day. I want to stay home with you.

After arranging to have her wait in the classroom to be picked up, and addressing the boy's foul language with the teacher, we found a way for her to change boring work to excellence by going the extra mile. We set up a reward system for achieving this by arranging trips together that she loves.

Listen to Messages About What Should be Healed Before Symptoms Appear

I believe in a gentle awakening from a night's sleep. It is, after all, the time to integrate the messages from the dream states that signal areas of concern[2] before they become disease symptoms.

It is a time for affection as a way of waking your child with gentle music and the question, "What did you dream?" Sometimes they do not feel like talking – which should be honored. They are still integrating the messages of the dream states.

Mornings can be hectic if we let them be or they can be a gentle making of our peace with a new day. We lay her clothes out the pre-

---

2 See Appendix II.

vious night. She chooses her clothes and I match her hair bands and, yes, even her underwear. This teaches her:
• That she dresses for herself, even though others cannot see;
• That her body is valued and celebrated through private ways;
• That elegance and grace of living means living deliberately and with extra care, rather than haphazardly.

I also have three highly successful, well-integrated adult children. They, as well as Jaylene, have always been given breakfast in bed. It is the easiest, least time-consuming way for me. It also allows them to stay in their 'cocoon' a little longer as they contemplate the day.

The affection you give by stroking their hair, massaging their back, kisses on the back of the neck, etc., penetrates through their defenses when they are half asleep (in the case of teenagers). Tell them why they are wonderful to have as a son or daughter.

It is often the flawed belief that when they reach puberty the parent should 'step back' from tactile affection – the very reason young adolescents often become promiscuous. The sudden withholding of affectionate touch can further add to their confusion as they deal with bodily changes.

The nature of touch can change throughout the years, but it should never go away. The healing power of touch should not be underestimated as you make it a point to:
• Hold your baby while bottle-feeding. Breast-feeding is of course infinitely preferable as it helps establish a healthy immune system;
• Make time for hugs when a child leaves or re-enters the house;
• Teach your child about love by being affectionate with your spouse or partner;
• Touch with love and gentleness areas of injury. Sing a soothing song to a little one's scuffed knee or bumped head.

And above all, be generous with your praise and gentle in correcting their behavior. This prevents their hiding their life from you in fear of being exposed to your criticism.

Touching Infants

- The bodies of babies become fatigued after their care has involved being picked up and put down throughout the day. The late afternoon is therefore the time they are most likely to be fussy. If you can, prepare family meals ahead and take the time to cradle the baby as you play soothing music, dancing slowly to its rhythms. This helps transition the baby to feeding and bath.
- The touch of water is reminiscent of the womb. Don't hesitate to do more than one bath a day. When the toddler stage is reached, bathing with you by candlelight can become a pleasant nightly ritual. My daughter took her first steps in the candlelit atmosphere of the bath, knowing the soft gravity of water and the close support of my body nearby. I have never used soap on her flawless skin, except for handwashing, and her body is virtually odorless. My own use of soap is likewise limited to my face and hands.
- Swaddling a baby simulates the secure confinement of the womb and lessens the overwhelming experience of exposure to life outside the uterus. Swaddling is a way of wrapping an infant so that their neck is supported and their arms and legs do not move about.
  - Place a cotton receiving blanket on a flat, soft surface such as a bed.
  - Fold one corner down where the baby's head is to be placed; the edge of the folded section will reach above the neck to slightly above the base of the skull.
  - Place the baby on the blanket as described.
  - Fold up the bottom corner of the blanket to cover the torso.
  - Fold over the sides one at a time, making sure the edges do not obstruct the baby's mouth.
  - The baby will now feel secure and can easily be carried without chafing its sensitive skin when being handled.

Nutritional Eating –
The Basis of Good Health

"The intelligent person, remembering the pain of diseases, should take food which is suitable to him and according to proper quantity and timing."
                    —*Charaka Samhita, Ayurvedic Medical Text*

NUTRITIONAL EATING

It is a cosmic law that you strengthen what you oppose – an important principle to remember when raising a child. Good nutritional habits are built not from what you tell them *not* to eat, but from what they grow to love from your cooking.

The same principle applies to other areas of your child's life. Opposing drug use does not take away the root cause. Whether it is addiction to food or drugs, any addiction comes from abandoning the self. When you encourage your child to listen to their dreams, their body signals, their hearts, they learn to live a life of authenticity. In touch with themselves, they have no need to reach out for something to fill a gap.

Many books are available on nutrition, but if your child has ever had a bout of antibiotics, the essential one is *The Body Ecology Diet*, by Donna Gates.

Nutritional Pointers

• Diet is crucial in treating teenager's acne. Avoid dairy, grease and fast foods. Getting children to drink enough water each day to promote proper elimination is not easy. Mint water with lemon is more attractive. Try chilled herbal tea sweetened with stevia drops (those that don't contain alcohol). Lymph flow is the key factor in clearing acne as well as the liver.[3]

• Finding a healthy sweetener is a core challenge of a good diet. We suggest liquid stevia or xylitol.

• Cow's milk, wheat and corn are the biggest offenders as far as food allergies are concerned. Eliminate them if the immune system seems stressed.

---

3 See www.belvaspata.com for a 5-month complete purification program that works wonders.

Natural Home Remedies

"Never put on a child's skin that which is not fit to take by mouth. The skin is our largest area of absorption. Read labels; some baby shampoos contain formaldehyde to prevent it stinging the eyes."

—Almine

"We shall seek temperance and a simple life. Real wealth and freedom consist in a minimum of needs."

—Epicurus

HOME REMEDIES

If you teach your child that the world around him is supportive and healing, you raise a self-reliant child. Children from 6 years to adulthood will benefit from the following books. You can read them to younger children.

- *The Vision*, by Tom Brown
- *Grandfather*, by Tom Brown

These books teach about the aliveness of all things and how we can be supported by cooperating with nature.

We can stock our homes with many natural remedies that abound in our physical environment. Some of them are described below.

For bites, stings and sunburn

- If you do not have an insect repellent handy that contains citronella oil, rub the outside surface of some orange peel across your child's exposed skin.
- Cut open an aloe vera leaf and apply the gel inside it to the injury. Aloe vera gel can also be purchased in a pharmacy[4] or health food store. Applying aloe vera after you have treated the bite or burn helps the skin to heal.
- Chilled witch hazel, white or apple cider vinegar also stops itching.
- Activated charcoal is another treatment for spider or other bites and stings. Remove any stingers first, however. Use clean water to make a paste of the charcoal and apply it to the affected area. A piece of plastic wrap covered with a bandage will keep the substance in place. This is also an excellent remedy for boils or pimples.
- A paste of baking soda and cool water is an excellent antidote for stings.

Note: if the sting creates an allergic reaction with abnormal swelling, difficulty in breathing, welts and signs of shock, call for emergency medical assistance immediately.

---

4 Rub a bit of the gel on your skin after cleansing at night for soft skin in days.

Burns

• Apply ice topically at once to stop further skin deterioration. The ice should remain in place for about 10 seconds; then wash the area with cool water in which tea (black/pekoe) has been steeped. The tea contains tannic acid, which heals burns[5]. Creams and ointments containing tannic acid can be applied to the burn before covering them with a gauze or bandage so that it does not stick to the burned area. As the burn begins to heal, apply pure lavender oil regularly twice a day to prevent scarring.

Diaper Rash and Other Skin Irritations

• Zinc ointment of any kind, under any brand name, will work overnight. Wash the affected area with cool water or cool calendula flower tea.[6]

Diarrhea

• Slippery elm power assists in regulating the bowel. Mix about a teaspoon of the powder into the baby's cereal. Use about two doses per day. Eliminate fruit juices and use rice or oatmeal to bind the bowel movements.

Constipation

• Some baby cereals, like rice cereal, can cause constipation as does insufficient water intake. Babies should have bottles of pure water as well as fruit juice and milk.
• A teaspoon of slippery elm powder mixed into fresh pear puree is also a valuable help.
• Older children can eat figs, prunes and real maple syrup.

---

5 Tannic acid powder dissolved in cool bath water alleviates sunburn.
6 Boil 1 quart of water and pour over 1 cup of calendula flowers. Let steep about ten minutes, strain and apply.

Food poisoning in older children

• Mix a tablespoon of apple cider vinegar (the cloudy type with the mother in it) in 8 ounces of water. The child should drink it all. Two capsules of food grade, activated charcoal should be taken with water twice a day.

Chest Congestion and Croup

• When a child has a croup-like, barking cough that is accompanied by wheezing and difficulty breathing, sit or stand in a steam room – or in a long, hot shower – while holding the child. The child should be able to inhale the steam but not come in contact with the water.
• You can also place a vaporizer inside a 'tent' created with blankets or plastic tablecloths around the child's head.[7]
• If the cough is unproductive and the chest congestion seems to be stuck, increase liquid intake. Use soups as well – onions and garlic are antiviral.
• Use the vaporizer and play the following game (best after a warm bath).
   ○ As the child lies face down, place pillows under the child's stomach and hips so they are elevated above the chest. The chest should be slanted downward.
   ○ With cupped hands and using an impact that is firm but comfortable for the child, sing a cheery song and play 'drum' on the child's back, always moving the impacts from the lower lung area toward the shoulders.
   ○ Do this for the time it takes to sing a few songs. It helps move the phlegm up so it can be coughed out.
• When a child resists herbs you wish to give him:
   ○ Place the herbs in a plastic bag and pulverize them with your fingers;
   ○ Remove the powdered herbs, mix them with a little almond oil to make a paste;

---

7 Do not leave small children unsupervised around plastic bags that could block air pathways.

○ Rub the paste on the soles of the feet;
○ Put cotton socks on the feet and have the child wear them overnight. Feet absorb a great deal.
○ This works best when the feet have first been soaked in warm water.

Colds

• A vaporizer in the room where the child is sleeping helps keep the congestion fluid.
• A dab of lavender oil on the pajama collar or top and a warm footbath with lavender oil in it is advised.
• The child should drink lots of freshly squeezed orange juice or orange juice not from concentrate.
• Camphor, mint and peppermint interfere with the working of any homeopathic remedies you may wish to use.[8]

Coughs

• For older children, give a tablespoon of equal parts lemon juice and honey mixed.
• In a health food store, find a good remedy that contains licorice or cherry bark.

Earache

• Earaches, chest congestion and sinus problems are frequently caused by dairy products. Goat's milk can often be tolerated when cow's milk cannot, as it is quite different and produces less mucous.
• When a doctor has checked that the eardrum is not ruptured, you can use almond or mullein oil that is warmed to just above body temperature. Place 3 drops into the infected ear, massaging lightly just below the earlobe.
• If the child who has an earache leaves the house, he or she should wear a knitted cap of some sort to keep the ear warm.

---

8 Honey should not be given to small children as it may carry the risk of botulism.

• If an insect has entered the ear, hold a light close to the ear for about 5 minutes. Attracted by the light, insects often move toward it. If this does not work, place 3-4 drops of almond oil in the ear, tilt the head toward the shoulder and place a white washcloth beneath the ear to catch the oil and, hopefully, the insect. If this does not produce the insect, consult a doctor.

• Excessive wax buildup can be produced in some children. For the very youngest, consult a doctor. For older teenagers you can buy ear candles. Always assist them when these are used (because of fire hazards) by carefully following the directions provided. Beeswax is antiseptic and the best.

Note: Almond oil is invaluable for many medicinal uses such as:

• Cleaning a little boy's penis under the (hopefully uncircumcised) foreskin.

Fever

• Fever of 101o or less requires heat and warmth: a warm bath; a hot water bottle at the feet (you want to draw the fever downward); a warm footbath with a tablespoon of Echinacea and liquid Vitamin C in it.

• Keep the patient warm and in bed, drinking lots of orange juice (diluted for children under five), fresh squeezed if possible or not from concentrate.

• An almond oil and Echinacea paste on the feet covered with cotton socks can be used.

• If the child has a higher fever, they need to be cooled. Never use alcohol on a child – it can induce hyperglycemia.

• Never put on a child's skin anything you would not give them by mouth; skin absorbs very well.

• To bring the high fever down, give the child a tepid sponge bath. Place a cool, damp washcloth on the forehead, replacing it every few minutes.

• Do not let them get chilled.

• If you are not able to bring down a fever of more than 101o in 20 minutes, consult a doctor.

- Fever is the body's way of fighting off germs. Do not be afraid of it but watch for dehydration symptoms such as:
  - When you pinch the skin together, it does not immediately return to its normal smoothness but retains the wrinkle for a while;
  - The amount of urination is at least half of what it usually would be;
  - The lips look dry and chapped;
  - Give room temperature fluids to a fevered child; they are apt to throw up chilled drinks.

Giggling incontinence

In the United States, 7% of pre-teen and teenage girls and 3% of boys in the same age bracket, suffer from this disorder.

- Try incontinence underwear so they will have less fear of an embarrassing incidence.
- Insist on regular and proper voiding – sitting up straight and taking their time.
- The most effective treatment may involve a simple trip to a very good chiropractor. Children often fall during play, displacing the sacrum where the nerves for bladder control originate.
- This can also become a problem with the onset of menstruation when the uterus swells.
- Strengthen the muscles by having the child practice cutting off the stream of urine mid-stream by contracting the muscles when voiding.

Head Lice

There are multiple known remedies for this highly contagious condition that spreads through schools.

- Lanolin packed into the hair and left overnight suffocates most lice.
- There are also various commercial remedies on the market. Herbal, non-toxic ones are preferable.
- Toys need to be tied in plastic bags and left for a few weeks so the eggs will hatch and die.

- Surfaces should be cleaned thoroughly and herbal solutions are available for this use.

There have been cases when, after trying everything, parents have considered the drastic measure of cutting the child's hair. I reached this point with my daughter's beautiful long hair when, as a final solution, she was given a permanent without using rollers to curl the hair. Not only did this completely deal with the eggs left in her thick hair but the smell of the solution that lingered for weeks prevented further infestation. The condition of the hair was restored with multiple deep conditioning treatments.

Influenza

- Oscillococcinum, a homeopathic flu medicine obtainable in health food stores, is an absolute must to have on hand. Follow instructions on the packaging and keep your child warm, avoiding any sudden temperature drops.
- Keep the diet light (soups, etc) and avoid mucous-forming foods like dairy or sugar.
- Give lots of liquids.

Indigestion

- Use peppermint tea for indigestion and tummy aches, ginger tea for nausea.
- Papaya or pineapple juice helps digest heavy meats.
- *The Body Ecology Diet* by Donna Gates has been an absolute mainstay in teaching principles of food combinations and how to restore the bodily terrain to one that is inhospitable to viral and bacterial infections, parasites and viruses - an absolute must for the parent of a child with chronic or regularly occurring conditions. We consider it normal for everyone to have colds, but it is not. In eleven years, my daughter Jaylene has had two rapidly passing, mild colds.
- The rules of thumb for good food digestion (undigested food becomes tomorrow's food allergies) are:

○ Replace dairy with unsweetened almond milk and sweeten it with stevia;

○ If you do use dairy, use it alone – it inhibits the digestion of other food;

○ Little children do not digest heavy oils well; even olive oil is too heavy. Use coconut butter (not oil) and ghee[9] for cooking. Use cold pressed flaxseed oil for salad dressings.

○ Do not combine fruit with any other food. Like milk, it should be taken alone.

○ Do not combine protein and carbohydrates

Inflammation

• Soak the area in a solution of water and Epsom salt or sea salt for 20 minutes.

• Pour a thick amount of castor oil onto a washcloth or piece of flannel (Edgar Cayce advises a piece of sheep or lambskin). Place on the affected area, heating the compress with a hot water bottle (an electric heating pad or blanket produces geopathic stress).

• Goldenseal powder mixed with almond oil can be used directly on the area, alternating with the castor oil packs, twice a day.

Infections of the Eyes

• Pink Eye, or conjunctivitis, creates abnormal redness in the eye, often accompanied by excretion of creamy, yellowish matter that glues the eyelashes and lids together. It is contagious and can spread from one eye to the other, so tell your child not to touch their infected eyes and to keep their hands clean.

○ To treat Pink Eye, boil enough water to ensure you have a full pint. Add and dissolve ⅛th teaspoon boric acid powder. Dip a clean white washcloth into the lukewarm solution and gently sponge the **closed** eye, carefully removing the crusted matter. Dip the washcloth into the solution only once and be careful not to contaminate it with your hands. Repeat every two hours.

---

9 Ghee is clarified butter made by boiling butter, letting it sit and then removing the milk solids that rise to the top when it has cooled.

Other Infections:

- Use the same method of sponging boric acid solution onto the area. If the skin is open or raw, seal it with aloe vera gel followed by a bandage.

Ingrowing toenails

Although this condition is usually found in adults, it can occur in children as well from the following causes:
- Irregular trimming of toenails;
- Irregular monitoring of shoe sizes. Growth spurts at times cause a skip in shoe sizes, so have them measured regularly;
- Pointed shoes, a fashion that comes and goes for teenagers;
- Incorrect trimming of toenails. They should be clipped straight across, not rounded like fingernails.

To treat this condition, create a tiny ball of cotton about the size of a grain of rice. Dip it in lavender oil and wedge it firmly under the in-growing corner of the nail. It may be a little uncomfortable, but will immediately provide relief from the edge of the nail that is growing into the flesh. It raises the nail enough to allow it to grow properly. Leave the cotton in place for about a week then remove.

Injuries, sprains, bruises and trauma

- Calendula tea dabbed or dripped into open wounds heals them quickly. Calendula ointment can also be used.[10]
- Arnica 30C is a handy remedy. It helps with any trauma suffered by the body and arnica oil is great for bumps and bruises.
- Washcloths soaked in cold apple cider vinegar or chilled witch hazel can be used for bruises and sprains. Headaches also benefit from application of a washcloth soaked in chilled vinegar.
- If a child has suffered shock, remember:
  - If the child is pale, raise the feet and legs;
  - If the child is flushed, raise the head;[11]

---

10 Also the boric acid solution mentioned under eye infections.
11 Memory clue, "If the child is pale, raise the tail. If the child is red, raise the head."

○ Keep them warm.
• Soak sprains, bruises and swelling in a solution of Epsom salt or sea salt. For baths, use a half cup of salt per gallon of water.

Nausea and vomiting

• Ginger is good for any nausea, even motion sickness.
• Bracelets can be purchased that have a bead positioned on the acupuncture point of the wrist that, when stimulated, prevents motion sickness.
• Chamomile tea helps calm the stomach.

Nosebleeds

• Phosphorous homeopathic remedy is commercially available. Keep it on hand if your child is prone to nosebleeds. It helps staunch other bleeding as well.
• While rocking the child in your lap, gently but firmly hold the bridge of the nose at the point just between the eyes. The child should be upright so that blood does not flow downward into the throat – which causes nausea.
• A washcloth dipped in ice water should be held on the upper lip and another placed on the back of the neck at the base of the skull.

Slivers/splinters and other foreign objects

• Silica 30C helps to expel foreign objects from the body in case you are unable to physically remove them.
• Otherwise, soak the area in warm water to soften the skin and remove the object with a sterilized needle or tweezers.

Sore throat

• Onion soup is helpful since it is antiseptic.
• For little ones, place Echinacea and almond oil on their feet to strengthen their immune system.
• Older children can gargle warm salt water (1 tsp to 1 cup of water).

- Make sure they drink lots of orange juice.
- Sugar inhibits the proper working of the immune system and dairy creates mucous. Eliminate these until the throat is healed.
- Zinc lozenges are also helpful.

Sprains

Sprained ankles and other joints can swell rapidly and may also discolor.

- Arnica 30C helps with shock.
- Soak the affected area in an Epsom salt solution for 15 minutes, then dab dry.
- Elevate the area if possible.
- Place washcloths soaked in ice cold apple cider vinegar on the area for 20 minutes. Dry and gently rub in arnica ointment.

Stomach ache

- Give peppermint tea to children over 5 years and place heat on the stomach.
- For infants, the warmth of your hand on their stomach is helpful.

Urinary tract infections

These are often the nemesis of little girls who take bubble baths. The alkalinity of the soapy bubbles destroys the acid mantle of the skin. It also irritates the genital membranes and disturbs the pH of the area.

- Cranberry juice several times a day and lots of water will help.

Warts

- The dandelions in your yard can take care of these. The white sap from the stem and root, dripped onto the wart every day, will usually clear it up in about 10 days.

THE HOME APOTHECARY

For those parents who want to learn energy healing for their family, see www.belvaspata.com. An offshoot of Belvaspata, Kaanish Belvaspata, has been reported to have miraculous effects in helping reduce tension and discord in families – a major cause of disease symptoms in children.

General Supplies

Bandages – different types
Bandaids – different types
Cotton balls & swabs
Cotton gauze
Cotton socks of the proper size (keep outgrown socks to use for herb pouches to put in bath water)
Earcandles
Enamel basin
Hot water bottle
White washcloths

Books

The Body Ecology Diet, by Donna Gates

Herbs

Calendula flowers, dried
Dandelion plants
Echinacea, powdered
Goldenseal, powdered

Homeopathic remedies

Arnica 30C
Oscillococcinum homeopathic remedy
Phosphorus homeopathic remedy
Silica 30C

Liquids

Cough medicine from a health food store
Echinacea
Witch hazel, refrigerated

Oils

Almond oil
Arnica oil
Castor oil
Lavender oil (Young Living Oil is excellent)[12]
Mullein oil

Powders and salts

Activated charcoal, powdered and capsules
Baking soda
Boric acid powder
Epsom salt

Salves, gels and ointments

Aloe vera gel (keep aloe vera plants as well)
Burn ointment containing tannic acid
Calendula ointment
Zinc ointment or diaper rash ointment containing zinc

Vitamins and minerals

Vitamin C with Echinacea
Zinc lozenges for sore throat

The kitchen pharmacy

Apple cider vinegar, the cloudy type, refrigerated
Prune juice
Raisins (shelf life 9 months)

---

12 To order, call 877 552-5646.

Real maple syrup
Stevia drops without alcohol

Teas

Breakfast tea bags for burns
Chamomile tea bags
Calendula tea (loose or in bags)
Peppermint tea bags

Reading Labels for Safety

The National Institute of Occupational Safety and Health Administration (OSHA) has identified 884 toxic or potentially cancer-causing agents in common personal care products. Of these, 778 were identified as causing acute toxic effects.

"Nothing in life is to be feared. It is only to be understood."

— Madame Marie Curie

THE ENEMIES IN THE BOTTLES

Identification of potentially cancer-causing agents in everyday, personal care products includes the following findings:
- 146 cause tumors, some of which are cancerous;
- 314 cause developmental abnormalities adversely affecting fetal development;
- 376 can cause eye and skin damage.

The FDA has no resources earmarked to assess chemical safety.

Dr. Samuel Epstein, Chairman of the Cancer Prevention Coalition and Professor Emeritus at the University of Illinois, has written more than 260 scientific articles and 10 books such as *Safe Shopper's Bible* and *Unreasonable Risk*. He has pointed out that incidence of childhood cancer has risen more than 35%. He says that cancer is mainly caused by chemical and physical agents in our environment and products.

The public is exposed to carcinogens in food, household products, cosmetics, PRESCRIPTION DRUGS and toiletries. Suggested reading: *Cosmetics Unmasked* by Drs. Stephen and Gina Antczak; *The Politics of Cancer Revisited* by Dr. Samuel Epstein and *Saving Face* by Dr. Sabina De Vita.

Dr. de Vita states: "Every time you reach for the bottle of fragrant shampoo, soap or cologne you are contaminating yourself and the environment. ... how sanitary is it to wash with engine degreaser or use antifreeze on your armpits and your teeth? Would you eat butylated hydroxytoluene (BHT) or stearamidoprophyl dimethylamine for breakfast? Most people do so without realizing it by the application of everyday toiletries on their skin. Your skin eats, too!"

Dr. de Vita continues in her book *Saving Face*. "There is evidence showing that the permeability of skin to carcinogens may be greater than that of the intestines. As presented at the 1978 congressional hearings, the absorption of nitrosodi-ethanolamine (NDELA) formed by nitrosation of DEA is over 100 times greater from the skin than by mouth.

Consumption of this carcinogen has been associated with up to 4- and 7-fold increased risk of childhood brain cancer and leukemia." (Dr. Epstein)

Some ingredients to immediately avoid

1. Alcohol - may increase the risk of tongue and throat cancer; contributes to hyperglycemia in children

2. Aluminum - is linked to nerve damage, breast cancer, Alzheimers

3. DEA (diethanolamine)/TEA - cancer-causing, found in many toiletries and cosmetics

4. Propylene glycol - carries a risk of kidney and liver abnormalities and skin cancer

5. Sodium Lauryl Sulphate – engine degreaser; found in shampoos that can affect development of children's eyes; so caustic that it causes eventual hair loss by damaging the hair follicle and impeding hair growth.

6. Toluene – an endocrine disrupter; may cause birth defects.

7. Talc – Epstein has found that frequent use of talcum powder dramatically increases certain cancers

8. Diazo-lidinyl-urea – a pesticide used as a cosmetic preservative

9. Methylparaben – often causes allergic reactions

10. Propyl-paraben – can cause skin reactions

"In a study at Bristol University of 14,000 pregnant women (WDDTY, Vol. 10) it was found that women exposed to aerosol deodorizer and air fresheners experienced headaches and depression and the babies suffered from ear infections and diarrhea. Unfortunately there is no regulation in the fragrance industry, even though chemicals in perfume are as damaging to health as tobacco smoke." *Saving Face*, Dr. de Vita.

> *"The sages follow the laws of nature and therefore their bodies are free from strange diseases. They do not lose any of their natural functions and their spirit of life is never exhausted."*
> —*Chinese Inner Classic*

READING LABELS ON FOOD
(Home-cooking of whole foods is always best)

Food Additives to Avoid (listed alphabetically)

Acesulfame K
Known commercially as Sunette or sweet One, acesulfame is a sugar substitute sold in packet or tablet form, in chewing gum, dry mixes for beverages, instant coffee and tea, gelatin desserts, puddings and non-dairy creamers. Tests show that the additive causes cancer in animals, which means it may increase cancer in humans. Avoid acesulfame K and products containing it.

Artificial colorings
The great bulk of artificial colorings used in food are synthetic dyes. For decades synthetic food dyes have been suspected of being toxic or carcinogenic and many have been banned. Whenever possible, choose foods without dyes. Natural ingredients should provide all the color your food needs. (FYI – the natural color of ripe oranges ranges from buttercup yellow through cadmium, depending on the variety and the soil in which the tree is grown. The brilliant orange color is a dye applied in wholesale packing houses. A ripe orange may display a tinge of green; ripeness is determined by sugar content.)

Aspartame
This sugar substitute, sold commercially as Equal and NutraSweet, was hailed as the savior for dieters for decades who had put up with saccharin's unpleasant aftertaste. There are quite a few problems with aspartame. The first is phenylketonuria (PKU). One of 20,000 babies is born without the ability to metabolize phenylalanine, one of the two amino acids in aspartame. Toxic levels of this substance in the blood can result in mental retardation. Beyond PKU several scientists believe that aspartame might cause altered brain function and behavior changes in consumers. And many people (though a minuscule fraction) have reported dizziness, headaches, epileptic-like seizures and menstrual problems after ingesting aspartame.

Avoid aspartame if you are pregnant, suffer from PKU or think that you experience side effects from using it. If you consume more than a couple of servings a day, consider cutting back. To be on the safe side, don't give aspartame to infants. Replace it with stevia.

BHA & BHT
These two closely related chemicals are added to oil-containing foods to prevent oxidation and retard rancidity. The International Agency for Research on Cancer, part of the World Health organization, considers BHA to be possibly carcinogenic to humans and the State of California has listed it as a carcinogen. Some studies show the same cancer-causing possibilities for BHT.

BHA & BHT are totally unnecessary. To avoid them, read the labels. Because of the possibility that BHT and BHA might cause cancer, both should be phased out of your diet.

Caffeine
Caffeine is found naturally in tea, coffee and cocoa. It is also added to many soft drinks. It is one of the few drugs – a stimulant – added to foods. Caffeine promotes stomach acid secretion (possibly increasing the symptoms of peptic ulcers) temporarily raises blood pressure and dilates some blood vessels while constricting others. Excessive caffeine intake results in 'caffeinism' with symptoms ranging from nervousness to insomnia. These problems also affect children who drink between 2–7 cans of soda a day. Caffeine may also interfere with reproduction and affect developing fetuses. Experiments on lab animals link caffeine to birth defects such as cleft palates, missing fingers and toes and skull malformations.

Caffeine is mildly addictive, which is why some people experience headaches when they stop drinking it. While small amounts of caffeine do not pose a problem for everyone, avoid it if you are trying to become or are pregnant. Try to keep caffeine out of your child's diet.

Note: Caffeine can be ingested in cases of severe migraine headaches to quickly relieve pain due to its dilating effects.

Monosodium glutamate (MSG)

Early in this century a Japanese chemist identified MSG as the substance in certain seasonings that added to the flavor of protein-containing foods. Unfortunately, too much MSG can lead to headaches, tightness in the chest and a burning sensation in the forearms and the back of the neck. If you think you are sensitive to MSG, look at ingredient listings. Avoid hydrolyzed vegetable protein, or HVP, which may contain MSG.

Nitrite and Nitrate

Sodium nitrite and sodium nitrate are two closely related chemicals used for centuries to preserve meat. While nitrate itself is harmless, it is readily converted to nitrite. When nitrite combines with compounds called secondary aminos, it forms nitrosamines, extremely powerful cancer-causing chemicals. The chemical reaction occurs most readily at the high temperatures of frying. Nitrite has long been suspected as a cause of stomach cancer. Look for nitrite-free processed meats - some are frozen as refrigeration reduces the need for nitrites – at some health food and grocery stores. Regardless of the presence of nitrite or nitrosamines, the high fat, high sodium content of most processed meats should be enough to discourage you from choosing them. And don't cook with bacon drippings.

Olestra

Olestra, the fake fat recently approved by the Food and Drug Administration (FDA) is both dangerous and unnecessary. Olestra was approved over the objection of dozens of leading scientists.

The additive may be fat-free but it has a potentially fatal side effect. It attaches to valuable nutrients and flushes them out of the body. Some of these nutrients – called carotenoids – appear to protect us from such diseases as lung cancer, prostate cancer, heart disease and macular degeneration. The Harvard School of Public Health states that 'the long-term consumption of olestra snack foods might therefore result in several thousand unnecessary deaths each year from lung and prostate cancers and heart disease and hundreds of additional cases of blindness in the elderly due to macular degeneration. Besides contributing to disease, olestra causes diarrhea and other serious gastrointestinal problems, even at low doses."

FDA certified olestra despite the fact that there are safe low-fat snacks already on the market. There is no evidence to show that olestra will have any significant effect on reducing obesity in America.

Despite being approved as safe by the FDA, all snacks containing olestra must carry a warning label (similar to the one found on cigarettes) that states:

> *This product contains olestra. Olestra may cause abdominal cramping and loose stools. Olestra inhibits the absorption of some vitamins and other nutrients. Vitamins A, D, E and K have been added.*

CSPI advises consumers to avoid all olestra foods and urges major food manufacturers not to make olestra-containing products.

Potassium Bromate

This additive has long been used to increase the volume of bread and to produce bread with a fine crumb (the non-crust part) structure. Most bromate rapidly breaks down to form innocuous bromide. However bromate itself causes cancer in animals. The tiny amounts of bromate that may remain in bread pose a small risk to consumers. Bromate has been banned virtually worldwide except in Japan and the United States. It is rarely used in California because a cancer warning is required on labels.

Sulfites

Sulfites are a class of chemicals that can keep cut fruits and vegetables looking fresh. They also prevent discoloration in apricots, raisins and other dried fruits, control 'black spot' in freshly caught shrimp and prevent discoloration, bacterial growth and fermentation in wine. Until the early 80's they were considered safe but CSPI found six scientific studies proving that sulfites could provoke sometimes severe allergic reactions. CSPI and the Food and Drug Administration identified at least a dozen fatalities linked to sulfites. All of the deaths occurred among asthmatics. In 1985 Congress finally forced FDA to ban sulfites from most fruits and vegetables. Especially if you have asthma, be sure to consider whether your attacks may be related to sulfites. The ban does not cover fresh-cut potatoes, dried fruits or wine.

Conclusion

Many packaged, canned and prepared foods contain food additives which help preserve the shelf life of the product. On average, a person consumes over 100 pounds of additives per year. Many, such as refined sugar, corn syrup, salt and MSG can have detrimental effects to your health. The most harmful are the ones chemically made by man. Your body has difficulty processing and eliminating them from your system. Therefore, some accumulate in your fatty tissues, leading to toxic reactions over time.

However, not all additives are toxic. Those made from wholesome, natural products are the least dangerous but intake should still be kept to a minimum. Below are lists of commonly used food additives. The first list contains generally safe additives and the second contains those that should be avoided. Both lists contain names typically found on food labels:

Generally safe to use

Annatto
Beet juice
Beet powder
Beta-carotene or carotene
Citric acid
Gelatin
Herbs and spices
Lactic acid
Lecithin
Minerals
Natural oils and extracts (e.g., almond oil, vanilla extract)
Natural sweeteners
Pectin
Sea salt

Natural rock salt
Sodium bicarbonate (baking soda)
Sorbic acid
Vegetable glycerin
Vitamins
Yeast

Ones to avoid

Aluminum salts
Artificial coloring
Artificial flavoring
Artificial sweeteners
Bisulfate
BHA
BHT
BVO
Caffeine
Carrageenan
EDTA
Hydrogenated oils
Metabisulfite
MSG
'Natural smoke flavor'
Olestra
Processed and refined sweeteners
Propylene glycol
Propyl gallate
Sodium benzoate
Sodium nitrate or sodium nitrite
Sulphur dioxide
THBQ

Developing Your Child's Inner Guidance

"Teach correct principles and as far as possible, let your children govern themselves."

—*Almine*

Knowing and not doing is equal to not knowing."
—*Chinese Proverb*

ENCOURAGING YOUR CHILD'S INNER GUIDANCE

A conversation with my daughter, Jaylene

J.: Mommy, are you the boss of me?

M.: You are the boss of you but I am the final authority. This means that if I see you lead yourself in the wrong direction I will step in and say 'No'.

J.: Why can you see the right direction and I can't?

M.: When one is watching each step you take on a path to make sure it's the right step, you may not notice that the path leads off a cliff. Even though the steps may be right, the direction may be wrong. I can see that at times when you can't.

J.: How can I be a direction-watcher and not just a step-watcher?

M.: By listening to your dreams. I'll show you how.

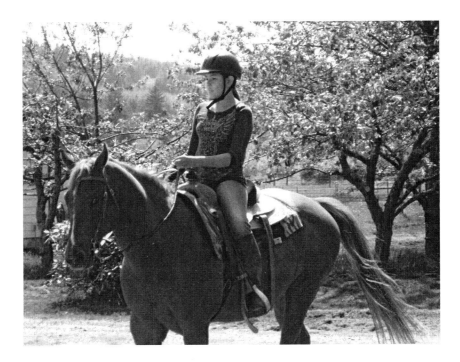

UNDERSTANDING YOUR CHILD'S DREAMS

EXCERPTS FROM THE MANUAL OF
SHRIHAT SATVA YOGA

Note: Shrihat Satva and Irash Satva Yogas are a wonderful way for children to release the messages of this and past life trauma that try to communicate with them through their dreams. Past lives – as well as birth trauma - are very fresh in their memories. My daughter spoke Anishabe, a Native American language, even though she had not been exposed to it in this life, and described her past life in great detail. She forgot the images of that life as she grew older. This is not uncommon in children. Whether suppressed into the subconscious or remembered, the hold of the past is presented for resolution in dreams.

Excerpt 1

In the practice of Shrihat Satva Yoga, multiple elements are combined to facilitate the removal of debris from previous incarnations.
• The musical elixirs used are an exact balance of black (subliminal) and white frequencies, utilizing the alchemical potencies of frequencies to balance out illusion. They form an essential component of this yoga practice.
• The Poetry of Dreaming is used to open non-cognitive communication with the deeper states of dreaming. This allows the issues of very old cycles of life to come to the surface for cancellation by the sound elixirs.
• The breathing rhythms and eye movement patterns of an individual reveal retained and suppressed trauma. Shrihat Satva Yoga uses these to trigger the release of debris from old incarnations.
• Shrihat Satva Yoga's postures frequently have the limbs crossing over one another. This is to facilitate merging the masculine and

feminine into the androgyny of enlightenment. They are also designed to open the gates of dreaming in the body.[13]

The human body is unique in that it is an exact microcosm of the macrocosm of created life. There are 12 points along the right, masculine side of the body and the same number on the left side. These are microcosmic replicas of the macrocosmic cycles of life.

The yoga postures are designed to open and remove the debris from these points – the gates of dreaming. This will occur physically through the postures and the music. Dissolving debris also occurs by way of dreaming (triggered by the breathing and eye movements), releasing past issues that caused the blockages in the points.

It is recommended that only a single verse be meditated on during a ten to fifteen minute period preparatory to commencing the yoga session. Have the meditation music playing 15 minutes before the yoga session to prepare the child as he sits quietly and meditating.

The music for this purpose is unique and irreplaceable for the purpose because it is sung in the old solfeggio scale. This is the scale used for Gregorian chants until it was banned by the Catholic Church in the early Middle Ages. Its effect of liberating the listener from belief systems is profound.

The yoga instructor should have the chosen verse accessible, either displayed in large letters or as a handout for the child.

The method is simple. The child reads the verse, empties his or her mind through entering a meditative state, and simply observes any images that arise and the subtle feelings they evoke.

During longer meditations this process should be done no more than three times in an hour. The child needs at least 10 minutes to rest and integrate the new qualities he or she feels within.

At no time should analysis be used. The more empty the mind, the more successful the non-cognitive communication from the deep psyche can be. Capturing in writing the images that arise can be helpful. Children should not think they have failed if in 15 min-

---

13 This form of yoga could be very beneficial for certain ADD and other behavioral disorders in children.

utes only a word is received. Different children may receive communications in different forms.

Note: The initial verse is like the end of a thread that is followed into the labyrinth of the deep chambers of the psyche. The images that arise from each 15-minute meditation are written down.

Excerpt 2

Cosmic cycles of life fall into two categories: those that can be called the ascension cycles and those that are called the descension cycles.

There are 12 electrical, masculine, light-based cycles; these are the ascension cycles. Likewise there are 12 cycles of a feminine, magnetic, frequency-based nature. Each of these has been repeated many times by all creatures as incarnation cycles.

The unresolved issues of those cycles, such as old belief systems, memories of pain and other distorted emotions are presented for resolution in dreams. There are 24 depths of dreaming, with the 12 more shallow ones communicating to us through dream symbols. The 12 deepest dream states are the feminine, non-cognitive states that cannot be interpreted through dream symbols and produce what to us seems like a deep, dreamless sleep. They speak to us through art and the Poetry of Dreaming.

This unique poetry communicates through omissions – that which is not said – imparting multiple depths of meaning revealing themselves as feelings and qualities. Although the Poetry of Dreaming uses literary devices such as assonance, alliteration, personification and sustained epithets, their use has profound purpose that transcends the obvious. The same applies to the use of adjectives in this type of poetry.

Its concise but powerful descriptive quality is reminiscent of the poetic form called Haiku, but whereas Haiku is bound by a rigid structure, the Poetry of Dreaming is not. Haiku provides the essence of simplicity that lies within the complexity of appearances. The Poetry of Dreaming whispers, through its rich imagery, of the primordial origins of the moment.

Yoga for Children

Shrihat Satva Yoga is more complex for little children as compared to Irash Satva Yoga. Yet it has been shown to yield the greatest results for ADD and other behavioral disorders. Visit www.yogaofillumination.com to learn how to do partial sessions for children.

Benefits of Shrihat and Irash Satva Yoga on Attention Deficit Disorder and Hyperactivity in Children and Adults

Although much research has been done to identify physical factors and causes contributing to Attention Deficit Disorder (ADD) and hyperactivity, very little has considered the element of spiritual causation. This lack of understanding is further exacerbated by associating these disorders within an 'umbrella' classification.

True Attention Deficit Disorder can be traced to several probable spiritual causes:

• **An advanced state of spiritual evolution**; The average man in the street lives in contracted awareness which allows him to focus on details. As he moves to the next evolutionary stage, that of the Master, his mind is silenced, he has no memory and exists in expanded awareness, unable to focus or retain even short-term memory.

• **Past life memory**; Time has lain like a spiral of black light and frequency behind the present life (white light). If a soul clings to past lives because of their glory or their pain, the soul force is mostly focused in those past incarnations, creating only a partial presence in the present. This results in a disassociated state.

The reality in which we live has had a parallel reality, also consisting of black light and frequency. Each of us has a presence consisting of multiple incarnations in both realities – like two ends of a stick. With two opposite poles, if one increases the other decreases. In the parallel reality consciousness is raised primarily through heightened frequency. Wherever polarity exists, one pole cannot be enhanced without reducing another. Therefore, if someone is a great Master in one reality, their light and mental abilities would be diminished in the other.

Attention Deficit Disorder

1. The music that is an integral part of both forms of the yoga incorporates the alchemy of sound. It uses the technique of precisely balancing black and white frequencies. In so doing the illusions of the past (and present) are cancelled out, releasing the energy and power that have been keeping these illusions in place.. That power and energy can then be used for the flourishing of the individual.

2. Shrihat Satva Yoga is designed to resolve the issues of prior incarnations, utilizing many methods including direct cognitive and non-cognitive communication with past lives. As it does so, the yoga practitioner becomes fully present in the moment with enough resources to raise his or her consciousness.

3. The gaining of resources in one reality, causing loss in another, is part of the illusion of separation. The practice of Irash Satva Yoga is designed to open gates in the body that access the endless supply of the Infinite's resources, allowing us to transcend the limited resources of polarity.

Hyperactivity

Hyperactivity can result from either or both of the following spiritual causes;

1. The person is in fact able to expand so much in consciousness that fear of their own vastness (and loss of touch with 'reality') catapults them into hyperactivity as preventive measure.

2. Their energy is so low that they attempt to produce more through frantic activity or cravings for foods or other substances to which they are allergic. This produces 'fake' adrenalin based on energy.

Other Benefits of the Yogas

The hyperactive adult or child could also be 'rushing away from' past trauma – even the trauma of birth – as well as suffering from the conditions described above. Resolving past issues and opening the gates of blocked resources should alleviate the condition.

There is a spiritual evolutionary stage beyond the over-polarization of the vast expansion of the Master and the over-contracted egotism of the fool. Both yogas are designed to elevate consciousness into more advanced stages. The stage of omni-perspectives lies beyond the expansion many are afraid of. It is a stage in which the individual can better function in the world while being free of the Dream.

Accessing The Messages Of The Dream Cycles

When the child wakes up, let it be a very pleasant experience. A rocking chair and soft music are helpful in not only calming a child before bedtime, but waking him or her from sleep. Encourage the child to share dreams. You can interpret the ones that are remembered according to the meanings given in Appendix I of this book. Use your common sense and the intuition parents are endowed with for those not listed.

The dreams not able to be interpreted in this way because they are not remembered in dream symbol imagery, need to be listened to in a different way.

1. Ask the child to paint you a 'word picture'.[14] You may have to give an example first, such as: "The little donkey stands in the golden twilight and watches the flight of swans leaving for winter."

2. Ask how his word picture makes him feel.

3. Pay attention to the feelings as well as the imagery. The symbols can be interpreted according to the dream symbols but the feelings constitute at least 80% of what the child is trying to say.

Examples Of Word Pictures

1. A luminous jellyfish, like a dilating sun, floats in the warmth of a boundless sea.

2. Laughter like soap bubbles floats on the air, tickling my nose, brushing my hair.

3. An antelope leaps under the all-seeing eye of the sun.

4. Through deep green moss the cool water drips across mountain crags.

5. Treasured dewdrop pearls strung on a spider web gently sway on the breath of the dawn.

---

14 *Labyrinth of the Moon* gives 144 such images as does Poetry of Dreaming in *Shrihat Satva Yoga*.

6. Water-lilies, floating in the silence of a moonlit pond, listen to the song of the night owl.

Helpful Hints to encourage Communication with the Deeper Psyche

1. If the child experiences a dilemma, have him or her ask themselves a question about the matter before they go to sleep. Upon waking, you follow four steps to elicit an answer:

    a. Ask "What do you feel or know about the question that you didn't know before?"

    b. If the answer has not presented itself, ask what dreams the child had. If there were some, interpret the symbols.

    c. If there were no remembered dreams, have the child paint a word picture and try to feel the answers it may be yielding.

    d. If this has not resolved the matter, ask your little one to remember anything special or unusual that happens in his day. Interpret this through dream symbols.

Further suggestions

1. The more you ask your child to feel the meaning of word pictures, the more adept he becomes in the language of the non-cognitive guidance of the psyche. The verses in *Labyrinth of the Moon* are archetypal. They represent the massive cycles of life (and incarnations) that mirror developmental stages found in the microcosm as well.[15] They assist communication with the 24 layers of the psyche and are beneficial to practice with – as a fun bedtime ritual, for instance.

2. Keep a journal in which your child's word pictures can go. Have him illustrate some or all. In our case, the interpretation of my daughter's drawings have yielded the most profound insights when other methods failed.

---

15 See *Journey to the Heart of God.*

TEACHING YOUR CHILD TO SEE BEHIND APPEARANCES

"The definition of a spiritual life is to see behind appear-ances. This is the first step in becoming free from the tyr-anny of form – which is mastery."

—*Almine*

Temper Tantrums

A temper tantrum is the outward expression of inner turmoil. It is therefore non-productive to take that outer expression at face value. Often the child directs the turmoil at a misperceived outer object – you, for instance, or another child touching his toy – not knowing why he or she is really angry.

The first thing to do is to give him space to calm down and come to terms with his feelings (the traditional time out). Do it in a non-punitive way by saying, "Go to your room". Or use the traditional standby, the water therapy bath with chamomile or lavender flow-ers tied in a cotton sock and hung on the running tap. You can then ask, "What is *really* bothering you? If you tell me about it, perhaps I can help.

An Example from my Daughter

J.: Stares furiously at me when I pick her up from school and mum-bles something I can't understand. She snaps at me when I ask what she said and goes to her room 'to be alone'.

M.: After an hour, I take her a snack. "You are unusually angry. What happened at school? Is it the rudeness of other kids? Did a teacher embarrass you or what? Tell me, problem-solving is my spe-cial talent and for your whole life I stand by your side."

J.: "The first one you said – about the rudeness", she mumbles from under her pillow.

Now that we have a starting point, I rub her back and get from her the story of who did what. Remember, insight yields positive emotions. I explain that a child screaming obscenities simply because she did not throw a stray ball back to him, is being spoken to like that in his home. We imagine what it would be like to live in that way and how future relationships will be for someone so dysfunctional.

Only after she's had her snack and watched a video, do I point out that in taking her hurt out on me in an angry way she is letting the obscene anger of the other child spill into our home life. We close the matter by agreeing that our home is the most wonderful place on Earth for us to be and that we do not live at the low level of treating each other disrespectfully.

Observations

1. No matter when you and your children unite after being apart, make time for their re-entry into the home. Only then is there a window of opportunity to hear about their day. They are never too old for this while they are in your home. This is especially important when young teenagers start to date.

2. Children learn most by example. It is your example of not engaging the superficial that trains them to live a spiritual life of depth. You cannot react in anger and then expect them to masterfully respond to life's circumstances. When you feel yourself slipping into frustration and anger, take 'time out' yourself before you respond. A bath works wonders for grownups too!!

3. It is essential for parents to schedule extra time for unforeseen crises with children – ("Oops, I have a school project due but I don't have the right materials!")as well as for – for nurturing moments and time to listen. It takes organization and discipline to run a household of peace and order, something that will be a gift to your family for the rest of their lives.

4. How did I know to guess that it was a child's rudeness that had angered Jaylene in the incident described above? She had dreamed that:

She was riding a bike down a hill where a group of boys asked her to ride back up the hill with them. At the top, their older brothers waited and tried to kidnap her.

Meaning: She went down to their level (riding down the hill) by acting as rudely as they. She brought them into her level (riding up the hill) by letting their rudeness spill into our home. Their family members held her captive, meaning that their influence seeped into our family and home and robbed her of her feelings of contentment and the freedom to enjoy the day.

Some hidden sources of children's anger

1. Acidic PH of the body: The result of stress; eating far too much starch and refined sugar; antibiotics.

2. A congested liver: The liver is the seat of anger in Chinese medicine. The condition can be caused by chemicals, food coloring, artificial flavors and refined sugar. The liver and gall bladder are paired organs. When one is in distress so is the other. The heavy fats of deep-fried foods, cheeses (pizza, etc.), canola and soy oils burden the gall bladder and back up the liver. Aspirin and other pain medications can cause permanent damage.

3. Allergies: They not only result from a congested liver but can cause that condition. They are primarily caused by vaccines, poor food combination (see Symptoms of Disease – Indigestion) and an overburdened immune system due to too many stressors in the environment. These stressors can come from fabric softeners, flame-retardant agents in clothing, perfumes in laundry detergent, shampoo, soap, pesticides in food, cooking in aluminum pots and other agents.

The spikes in adrenalin in the blood caused by allergens can cause a child to go into a state of emergency.

4. Candida Albercans: The condition of systemic fungal overgrowth is such a serious problem that it will take a very concerted effort by the whole family before it is conquered. It is the beginning of a breakdown of organ function (causing allergies, congested liver and gallbladder and an acidic PH which predisposes one to parasites, bacteria and viruses). The fungal overgrowth in the bowel is frequently caused by steroids, antibiotics and birth control pills. (See www.belvaspata.com for a 2-hour audio presentation on How to Heal Chronic and Systemic Diseases.)

The child with this condition will have raging emotions, inability to concentrate and continual physical ailments. The resulting impaired lymph flow brings skin outbreaks of various kinds, including acne. The buildup of toxins produces obesity, a growing problem among young people.

Candida symptoms
- abdominal gas and bloating
- headaches
- migraines
- excessive fatigue
- cravings for alcohol
- anxiety
- vaginitis
- rectal itching
- cravings for sweets
- inability to think clearly or concentrate
- hyperactivity
- mood swings
- diarrhea
- constipation
- hyperactivity
- itching
- acne
- eczema
- depression
- sinus inflammation
- pre-menstrual syndrome
- dizziness
- poor memory
- persistent cough
- earaches
- low sex drive
- muscle weakness
- irritability
- learning difficulties
- sensitivity to fragrances and/or other chemicals
- cognitive impairment
- thrush

- athlete's foot
- sore throat
- indigestion
- acid reflux
- chronic pain

CANDIDA ALBERCANS, THE SECRET EPIDEMIC

By Almine Barton, Jr., L.Ac, C.F.T.

One of the most important things to remember about Candida is that it can be cured. It may take serious commitment and perseverance, but it can be overcome and health restored. Many become very discouraged when they are told they have Candida Albercans, due to the fact they will have to make a drastic lifestyle change. People in the American culture are used to instantaneous cures. This mindset of fast and easy has become the downfall of the American healthcare system. It is, in fact, this consciousness that has created the epidemic of Candida in the first place through the use of 'miracle cures' like antibiotics and birth control pills. These detrimental medications not only feed Candida, but also create an environment conducive to harboring parasites.

One has only to examine certain words within the Western medical system to decode what they truly do to the body. Take, for instance, the word 'antibiotic'. Its literal meaning is 'anti-life'. Is this something we want to take into our body for healing? Birth control pills are another culprit. These pills are often given to girls in their teens, not only for prevention of pregnancy but also for regulation of menstruation and suppression of acne. The side effects range from dark circles under the eyes to flatulence, decreased immune function, compromised digestion, yeast infections, bloating, back pain and easy bruising. Some of the long term effects can include illness as serious as breast cancer.

Refined, non-organic foods are a major feeder of the overgrowth we call Candida. Refined foods are processed to the point where there is no 'chi' or life force left in them. These are the foods that the majority of Americans consume – dead food. Death can only create death and life can only create life. It is absolutely vital that the American public become educated in the importance of living foods, or foods containing live enzymes.

Vegetables, sprouts, grains, herbs, edible flowers, certain dairy products and krauts are just a few of these life-promoting foods. Refined foods contain no enzymes of their own, hence the growing need to ingest digestive enzymes with meals. Living foods contain their own enzymes necessary to break them down.

To eat organic food is highly desirable. First of all, by eating organically we support smaller local farms that provide an income for a family through ecologically sustainable and health-conscious methods of farming. These families work in harmony with the elements of our Earth. They do not use chemical pesticides or fertilizers that damage the fragile ecosystem of our world. These synthetic toxins also seep into groundwater and poison it to the extent that many people each year (yes, even in America) die from polluted water. Statistics show that the bee pollination of flowers rapidly declined in the 'bread basket' area of the Midwest United States. Why? Because the pesticides used on the crops affected the attraction of the bees to the local flora. By buying food that is not grown organically, we perpetuate environmental damage as explained in the previous examples.

Dr. Gabriel Cousins reports the following information in his book *Conscious Eating*: "The overall estimate of the Rutgers University research suggested that organic foods had 87% more minerals and trace elements than non-organic food that was commercially grown." He goes on to state: "The Firman-Bear report on research done at Rutgers University indicated that organically grown foods were much richer in minerals than the 'look-alike' commercial produce. For example, organic tomatoes had more than 5 times the calcium, 12 times the magnesium, 3 times the potassium, 600% more beneficial organic sodium, 68 times more manganese and 1900 times more iron than non-organic tomatoes."

Other statistics that resulted from the Firman-Bear study conducted at Rutgers University are:

1. Organic spinach had more than double the calcium, 5.5 times more magnesium, more than 3 times the potassium, 75 times the beneficial sodium, 117 times more manganese and 83 times the iron than that of non-organic spinach.

2. Organic lettuce had 3.5 times the calcium, 3 times the magnesium, 3 times the potassium. 33 times the beneficial sodium, 169 times the manganese and 57 times the iron than that of non-organic lettuce.

3. A Harris poll showed that 80% of Americans want organic fruits and vegetables and more than 50% are willing to pay the small added cost of buying organic.

People dealing with an immune disorder like Candida need all the nutrition they can get because they are nutritionally deprived. There are several reasons.

1. Their pancreas-spleen organ is not manufacturing enough digestive enzymes to digest food properly, so the Candida patient can feel they're not getting enough food, manifesting as a starving feeling inside.

2. Their colon walls are usually caked with putrefied foods that did not digest properly. This can cause bloating, enlarged abdomen, gas and constipation. The human body absorbs the nutrients, vitamins and minerals from food through the colon walls so if the colon is not completely clean and free of parasites or yeast, health problems persist.

Organic foods have more nutrition, which helps the body feel full and thereby prevents the starving feeling and lessens cravings. They also have more fiber and nutrients that push fecoid mucus matter, parasites and yeast out of the colon.

For these and many other reasons it is important that people eat organic foods.

Antibiotics and growth-promoting hormones are also in non-organic dairy, meat and egg products. These are fed to the animals to unnaturally produce more milk, become fatter for meat or to promote the animal's hormones to reproduce at a faster rate. So even if a person is not taking antibiotics or hormones but continues to eat non-organic dairy, eggs or meat products, they will ingest these substances through their food. Many scientists now believe that children exhibit more adult-like features at an earlier age due to the fact that they have grown up on a diet of antibiotics and growth hormones via their food. Remember, pesticides, growth hormones, toxic chemical fertilizers and antibiotics are all contained in the typical hot lunch meal served in school cafeterias.

Some other helpful tips for the person recovering from Candida:

1. Get a colonic once a month. Colonics are administered by a certified colon hydro-therapist. Many of these therapists have backgrounds in nursing and/or holistic Western European medicine such as homeopathy. Colonics were a vital part of European medicine for centuries and still are in many places around the world.

2. Acupuncture is immensely helpful in healing the body of Candida. The licensed acupuncturist can provide a vast resource of knowledge regarding human physiology. A practitioner of Chinese medicine will help the Candida patient by administering acupuncture for a 'damp spleen-earth' condition in the body. According to Ayurvedic, Tibetan and Chinese medicines, Candida is an excess of dampness and cold in the body's system. This assessment makes sense when you realize that yeasts and molds can only grow in a damp environment. The Ayurvedic physician would call this an excess of 'Kapha', while some Chinese nutrition consultants call it an excess of 'Chong'. A typical acupuncture treatment for the client dealing with Candida might entail acupuncture needles inserted into the points for spleen-pancreas, colon and/or liver. All of these organs closely affect one another in the domino-like breakdown of a Candida takeover in the body. In other words, because the pancreas does not have enough enzymes to break down the food, the food will rot in the colon and cake its walls. This will cause constipation, leading to a backed-up liver that cannot release its bile into the colon. So a knowledgeable acupuncturist would treat all of the above-mentioned organ points.

3. Large doses of pro-biotics such as L.Acidophilus, Bifidobacterium and FOS (fructooligosaccharides) re-plant healthy bacteria in the intestinal tract and colon, helping to eradicate Candida. The following excerpt is taken from the column "Frontiers of Science" in the January 1999 issue of Better Nutrition.

"There is a particularly good reason to supplement your diet with pro-biotics. We are facing a serious threat to public health today due to the overuse of antibiotics during the last 30 years. We have created 'super germs' that are drug resistant and impossible to restrain. Antibiotics not only destroy the good bacteria in the intestines but foster the ability of harmful strains to get a foothold. Keep in mind that even if you rarely medicate with antibiotics you are still exposed to them second-hand via non-organic meat and dairy products. Antibiotics upset the intestinal ecosystem. Since the digestive process is compromised, nutrient absorption is also suppressed and either constipation or irritable bowel syndrome may develop."

4. The fourth tool to help eliminate Candida is the use of apple cider vinegar. Many Candida diets prohibit any vinegar; however there is one kind of vinegar that does not feed the yeast but actually kills it and this is vinegar from apples. There are several criteria for true apple cider vinegar:

- **a.** It must be raw and unfiltered;
- **b.** It must be aged in wooden, not metal, barrels (metal breaks down the beneficial bacteria);
- **c.** It must contain 'the mother', or the beginning culture strain.

If it is true apple cider vinegar, you will see the culture floating around in murky bits and pieces within the liquid. Oddly enough, this is precisely why most Americans will not buy the true vinegar because it looks 'dirty'. This sediment is actually what the body needs to restore a healthy interior ecosystem.

Apple cider vinegar has been used for centuries as a folk remedy. It has been proven to help the following ailments; arthritis, colitis, dandruff, diarrhea, food poisoning, inflammation of the kidneys, obesity, insomnia, chronic fatigue, migraines, high blood pressure, dizziness, sore throat, over-sensitive eyes, impaired hearing, ear discharges, blocked nose, tickling cough, hiccups, hay fever, laryngitis, mild asthma, tooth decay, mouth ulcers, bleeding gums and fragile fingernails.

A wonderful food for pets is a tablespoon of flaxseed oil with 2 tablespoons of apple cider vinegar. Their urine will be rid of odor, their coats will shine, they will recover more quickly from illness and maintain a healthy weight.

Douching with apple cider vinegar will help rid a woman of yeast and bladder infections. It will also help counter toxic shock syndrome created by the unnecessary use of tampons.

5. Pre-digested foods are a must in the process of healing Candida. The reason many Asian people have longer lives and better health is because their diet contains sea vegetables, kim chee, krauts and kefir. Kim chee is a spicy type of kraut that is a staple in Korea, Vietnam, Laos, Thailand and parts of China. The old farmers of the Appalachian mountain range in America, particularly documented in Vermont, have been shown to outlive other populations in the United States. This is attributed to their diet which contains kraut, apple cider vinegar, honey, tubers, edible flowers, berries and vegetables. Pre-digested foods are exactly that, pre-digested, therefore the digestive process is made easier in the body because it does not have to do so much work. Kefir is another pre-digested food that is a favorite among the long-lived centenarian peoples of the Hunza Valley, Georgia, Ukraine and the Vilcbamban valley of the Andes. All of these locations have shown the highest populations of people that not only live well over 100 years of age, but thrive. They are still able to walk up and down the mountains, work in their gardens and procreate. For an interesting study of this, including photographs, see books on the Hunza Valley.

6. Sea vegetables are a wonderful addition to any meal. They are so packed with nutrients such as iron and B-12, that our culture would greatly benefit from taking notice of them. Unfortunately, most Americans seem to ignore them because we associate them only with Asian cuisine. What many people of European ancestry do not realize is that the Celtic, Pict, Norse, Germanic and Anglo-Saxon tribes of Europe thrived on sea vegetables as staples in their diet. To this day the seafaring folk of Ireland, Scotland, Wales and the British Isles still make their famous seaweed soup as shown in the movie "The Secret of Roan Innish".

These wonderful vegetables provided by the ocean are loaded with calcium and are nourishing to the thyroid, typically a problem with Candida-afflicted people. The Chinese physician would prescribe them nutritionally to someone with Candida because of the sea vegetable's ability to thrive in damp and cool environments like the ocean, reflective of the 'damp spleen-earth' condition within the body.

Sea vegetables also have an anti-radiation effect on the body. This means that for those exposed to a lot of radiation from computer screens, microwaves, appliances and televisions should eat them because they carry radiation and heavy metals out of the body.

7. The introduction of the stevia plant is nothing short of a gift to the sugar-infested West. This herb grows in the Andean foothills in Peru, Ecuador, Brazil and Paraguay, although it is most typically harvested in Paraguay. It is completely safe for diabetics because it does not raise blood sugar levels. It actually inhibits tooth decay, has virtually no calories, is packed with vitamins and nourishes the pancreas. It also takes care of the sugar cravings that the yeast perpetuates within the body.

It is so extraordinarily sweet that it is 200-300 times sweeter than white sugar! One-fourth of a teaspoon of stevia equals a half-cup of white sugar in sweetness. This also puts it at the most economic sweetener around because a little goes a very long way. Stevia is also heat stable, which makes it ideal for baking. It is used widely in Israel, China, South America and Japan (which imports the greatest volume). These countries use stevia as the main sweetener for toothpaste, bubble gum, and some candies. In Tokyo many restaurants have little packets of stevia on the tables for added sweetener just as restaurants in American have packets of Sweet n' Low on their tables. Sweet n' Low is not advised as a sugar substitute. The indigenous Guarani tribe of Paraguay has successfully used the stevia leaf and its flowers in a tea concoction for treatment of diabetes.

8. Warming, heating herbs are necessary to counteract the damp-coldness of the Candida-afflicted body. A Chinese or Ayurvedic physician would prescribe herbs that balance the dis-ease within the body. If the body is considered too 'yin', which it is when it has Candida, a Chinese physician would prescribe more 'yang' or warming herbs to bring balance to the body's ecosystem. Such herbs would include ginseng (American and Siberian), cayenne, garlic, lapacho (Pau d'arco), turmeric, hingwastaka, curry, cumin, astragalus, paprika, coriander and many others. These bring heat to dampness and warmth to the digestive tract, causing the digestive fire or 'agni' as it's called in India, to help break down the food better. These herbs also help peristalsis, which promotes the easy breakdown of proteins – a typical problem for people with Candida.

A patient with Candida may feel overwhelmed by the amount of information currently available on the subject. This is actually a positive thing. More and more people are becoming aware of the gigantic effects this secret epidemic is having on the world. Because public interest is growing, there are many books and diets available to the public. I have tried many different Candida diets and programs but none of them compare to the program called *The Body Ecology Diet* by Donna Gates. This book is an invaluable resource and the program will reverse even the most difficult case of Candida. I used this program for almost a year and a half. I shed 55 pounds, rid myself of yeast infections and no longer suffer from panic attacks, dizziness, loss of memory, flatulence, water retention, bloating, halitosis, rashes, loss of sex drive and other symptoms I had before starting the program.

Donna Gates has woven together the traditions of macrobiotics, food combining, eating according to blood type, juicing and detoxification into a cohesive program that contains benefits from many philosophies. To obtain a copy of *The Body Ecology Diet* or any of her other books such as *The Stevia Story* or *The Magic of Kefir*, visit her website at http://www.bodyecologydiet.com.

It takes courage to want to heal Candida. The process brings up very intense feelings with the 'die off' reaction of yeast eradication. It is imperative that one is surrounded by a loving, supportive and nurturing environment in order to heal the body with the maximum amount of support. This may require making some drastic changes within the household. The family of the patient with Candida needs to realize that the old way of eating, preparing and viewing food is past. It no longer applies. They need to show their support by not bringing sweets, poorly combined foods or anything not on *The Body Ecology Diet* into the house. This kind of drastic shift in a household can bring about positive changes for the entire family. Now that one person in the house is eating properly combined, wholesome, nourishing meals it is easier for other people to make a dietary lifestyle change.

The family will also need to support the use of chemical-free household cleaning supplies. People with Candida are extremely sensitive to aromas and chemicals. Not only does tobacco smoke bother them, chemical cleaners such as laundry and dish soaps have the potential to cause allergic reactions in the individual. Besides the fact that non-biodegradable household products are not good for our exterior environment, they are also not good for the body's inner environment. What damages the Earth damages our bodies.

An individual who has Candida is blessed in a way. I know that can be difficult to perceive, but one can view it in the light that people who have Candida actually become so refined intuitively to all that is not natural that their body actually rejects it. It one is committed to healing their Candida, then even through the darkest moments – and there will be some, they can safely assume their body will grow in health every day.

The body that is healing is able to tolerate more and more of Mother Nature's foods that are pure and natural even though the die off symptoms of the first three months on the program are very difficult. Perseverance, prayer and encouragement from the family will help the patient create a change in their digestion and absorption of foods. They will feel happier, more clear and better able to function and thrive.

I am not promising that major emotional trials will not happen. Every organ, according to Eastern medical philosophies, has a primal emotion associated with it. As we clean our bodies of the yeast, chemicals and toxins, each of the emotions will emerge to be faced. Each organ in a sense is a temple, isolating a certain emotion for the initiate to master.

Gregg Braden, geologist, author and lecturer mentions in his books *Awakening to Zero Point* and *Walking Between the Worlds* that the temples along the Nile River in Egypt were actually temples where a particular emotion was faced by the initiate. The Nile

River represented the spine, while each temple along it represented a chakra or energy center in the body.

You are to be congratulated for beginning the amazingly empowering process of healing Candida. I remember the first day in November 1998 when I had a bite of my first fruit in almost a year. It was like ecstasy. When one hasn't eaten a fruit in nearly a year, it is a heavenly experience and you realize what you have taken for granted for so long. Candida helps you begin to appreciate the natural sweetness in what Mother Nature provides. When you realize that the fundamental six tastes (mentioned in Eastern medical philosophy) are contained in all natural foods, you never have sugar cravings again.

Wellness is mankind's birthright. You have decided to claim it for yourself and your family by taking control of your health and stating to the yeast and parasites that your body is not their dwelling place. It is your temple and you have every right and obligation to keep your temple clean so the deity within it, your heart, may be in joy with the ecstasy of being alive.

This is a supportive and loving universe and world. Enjoy it.

The Sanctuary of Nature - Finding Solace for the Soul

"Many do not seek out the healing pristineness of nature, fearing they may be bored. But it is not boredom they fear, but silence. It is in the silences of our lives where we encounter ourselves."

—Almine

"Now I see the secret of the making of the best persons; it is to grow in the open air and to eat and sleep with the Earth."

—Walt Whitman

SEEING BEHIND APPEARANCES IN THE ENVIRONMENT

"There is no enslavement as complete as that created by social conditioning. The 'wisdom' of the parents cannot apply to the groundbreaking newness of the moment in a cosmos where nothing is as it seems. It but serves to bind the next generation's wings, preventing them from rising above the mediocrity of yesterday."

—Almine

It is an exceptional child who is literate in communicating with the world around him. The environment, just like our bodies and our dreams, conspires to guide us into cooperation with life's flow. It is only when we allow life to guide us through its gentle whispers, rather than its hard knocks, that we achieve a life of peace and radiant health.

The comfort of one's own company and the vital need for imaginative play and silence reveals guidance in that the child can puzzle out and come to terms with events in their life. This allows for the integration of experience and prevents the deafening dialogue of the mind found in most adults. The internal dialogue is man's coping mechanism for suppressing un-integrated experiences that have not yielded their insights.

But how does a child begin to puzzle out his world? By gradually learning to watch for notable events and then translating their meaning through dream symbols. But though this is a way of receiving information, life requires reciprocity.

Indigenous people have for eons known that life thrives from appreciation, whether it is a child or a plant. Tokens of love, praise and gratitude were left in the forms of tobacco, cornmeal, cocoa leaves, etc. It also is the foundation of the law of increase. Having your child find one thing daily for which to be grateful and teaching him or her how to express their thanks is a good way for them to learn that behind the appearances of separation lies the interconnectedness of life.

When my three oldest children were growing up, their friends would come for dinner and some would end up staying from a few months to a few years, depending on factors in their families. Unlike other households, we had no television, video games or much in the form of electronic entertainment other than carefully chosen videos.

The absolute salvation for our household at that time was the introduction of these young teenagers to Tom Brown's books, *The Vision* and *Grandfather*. These are true tales of the education of Tom Brown and another youngster under the tutelage of Grandfather Stalking Wolf during their childhood. The discovery of the aliveness of all things through the pages of these books changed all our lives.

Their subsequent desire to enter nature, not as a visitor but as an interconnected part of it I supported wholeheartedly and the adventures began. I was a single mother at the time, as I am today, and earning a living combined with managing a bulging household got me into the wonderful habit of starting my day at 5:00 – 5:30 a.m. I realized that doing work as an act of devotion, with love, praise and gratitude in my heart meant that I did not tire, needed less sleep and had uninterrupted hours of fruitful organization and preparation.

Many wonderful nature experiences and many backpacked picnic lunches later, many of these young people left, never to return. But wherever they are they are listening to music that feeds the soul instead of heavy metal that breaks down the cells or other music with demoralizing lyrics.

Finding the silence

- Noise pulls us out of the moment – the place where all self-empowerment lies – and into the next. The noise pollution on the planet is a much overlooked factor in mental disorders and disease. Cancer, for instance, is a lack of presence. How can you be present for yourself when you are not living in the moment – the only place where self-connection takes place?

• Get rid of noise such as heating systems, freezers, etc., as much as you can and find the silence of nature often. Do not let TVs remain on when no one is watching.

• Mental silence is achieved by being in peaceful surrender to life and in touch with the stillness within. The constant states of emergency our young people are exposed to through electronic games, movies, and TV in general create high adrenal levels which in turn affect the blood sugar. This eventually leads to adrenal fatigue and the de-sensitizing of the child, who becomes unable to hear or appreciate the birdsong at dawn. Loud, blaring music has been shown to damage their hearing. The images on a flat screen likewise affect their depth perception.

Note: Parents seem to think at times that it is cruel to single their child out; to deprive him or her from what their peers are experiencing. But isn't that the very basis of preparing your child for an exceptional life; to soar unafraid like the eagle wherever your heart leads, without the shackles of another's approval? I explain to Jaylene why others seek constant electronic stimulation and why we do not: we explore life. She feels privileged, not deprived.

• Subliminal noise arises from geopathic stress and is a hostile and invasive waveform that produces cancer in rats. All electronics produce geopathic stress. Chunks of black tourmaline stone have been found by Dr. Robert Jacobs to help lessen geopathic stress when placed around televisions, refrigerators (they produce one of the highest levels of geopathic stress in the household). Sheets of cork placed under the mattress help insulate your little ones from geopathic stress coming from the wiring in floors and from underground streams.

We are just beginning to understand 'black noise' (irregular waveforms) and 'black sound' (regular waveforms). To use black sound as a tool to promote health, purification and enlightenment, see www.angelsoundhealing.com for a complete explanation and a sound-healing method you can use for your family.

GEOPATHIC STRESS
by Dr. Robert Jacobs, MRCS, LRCP

Frequently asked questions about geopathic stress

What is geopathic stress?

The term geopathic stress refers to the adverse effects on health of electromagnetic radiation coming from the earth. Scientific research, carried out mainly in Germany, has shown that some people's health is affected in a detrimental way by electromagnetic radiation coming from the earth itself where they live.

The most usual cause of geopathic stress is underground water, usually an underground stream, flowing beneath a house. The water rapidly flowing through rock gives rise to an electrical field which can affect the health of those living above it.

Geopathic stress can also arise from a geological fault line, that is, a deep crack in the bedrock which allows radiation from deep within the earth to come up to the surface. This too can affect the health of those living above a fault line.

Are there other types of geopathic stress?

Yes. These are due to the fact that the magnetic field of the earth is non-uniform. In other words, it is stronger in some places than it is in others. If the strength of the earth's magnetic field is measured on the ground using instruments such as magnetometers, it is found that it forms lines of force. These lines of force form a rectangular grid. This looks very similar to the liens of latitude and longitude on a map. This grid of lines of magnetic force is called the Hartmann Net.

If one is living in a house situated where the lines of force of the Hartmann Net cross each other, this may give rise to geopathic stress.

Measurements of the earth's magnetic field show also that there is a second grid system laid over the top of the Hartmann Net. This is known as the Curry Grid. Here the lines of force meet at an angle giving rise to a diamond shaped pattern looking rather like the pattern of an old fashioned leaded window.

The Curry Grid seems to give rise to more geopathic stress than does the Hartmann Net. Both can interact with each other and with stress coming from underground water and fault lines.

Of all the types of geopathic stress, that caused by underground water and fault lines is the most important.

Why is geopathic stress important and what effects does it have?

Geopathic stress can adversely affect the health of those whose houses are affected by it and it can be one of the many causes of chronic ill health. Fortunately its effects can be removed or neutralized (this will be discussed below).

Geopathic stress was first discovered in the 1920s by German doctors who were investigating cancer clusters. They were trying to find out why certain villages and streets in Germany had an unusually high incidence of cancer among those people living in them. They looked at all sorts of different factors without finding the answer. Finally, with typical German thoroughness, they looked at geology and found that the areas where there was lots of cancer all lay on geological fault lines. This led to the discovery of geopathic stress.

As geopathic stress is associated with an increased incidence of cancer it is something that needs to be taken very seriously indeed. However this does not mean that everyone who is geopathically stressed will get cancer. It is only one of many factors which predispose to the disease.

In my own practice I find that the main effect of geopathic stress is that it stops patients getting completely better. It appears to block the action of virtually any type of therapy. When patients tell me that they have already seen two homeopaths, an acupuncturist, and three Harley Street consultants, none of whom could get them better, I find that they are usually suffering from geopathic stress. I suspect that geopathic stress is the only reason for natural remedies to fail. If a patient does not respond to correctly administered remedies, and assuming that the disease is potentially treatable, one usually finds they are suffering from geopathic stress.

The reason for this appears to be that it continually disrupts the body's electrical field and its electrical control systems.

How can I tell whether I am affected by geopathic stress?

There are a number of pointers which may suggest the presence of geopathic stress by its effect on both people and buildings. The following clues may suggest that a person is affected by geopathic stress:

1. They have a serious illness such as cancer, M.E. or multiple sclerosis;

2. They have any illness which does not clear up despite good treatment;

3. They have tried a number of different therapies without success;

4. They feel better when away from home. For instance, a condition may clear up or improve when away on holiday only to come back again when they return home;

5. They become ill shortly after moving house;

6. They live in a house which has never 'felt right' or they instinctively dislike it;

7. They wake up feeling un-refreshed or feel worse in the mornings. This is because people are often affected by geopathic stress in bed as the body's resistance to it drops to a third of normal during sleep.

There are other pointers which may suggest that a particular house is affected. These are:

1. There may be problems with mold in the house;

2. There is a lot of lichen or moss growing on the roof, walls or lawn as geopathic stress encourages the growth of these;

3. There may be problems with ants, wasps or bees. Most animals avoid geopathic stress. Those that avoid it include dogs, cows and horses. Some are attracted to it and these include ants, wasps, bees and, oddly enough, cats;

4. The presence of cracks in walls, driveways, paving stones, kerbstones and roads. These may indicate the presence of a geological fault line;

5. The presence of trees with cancer, i.e., large knobbly growths on the trunk, or trees whose trunks have split into two;

6. Gaps in hedges. These may indicate the position of a line of geopathic stress crossing the hedge;

7. Close neighbors may also be in poor health;

8. The presence nearby of springs and wells;

9. Previous occupants of the house have also been ill.

Geopathic stress is far more frequent where the water table is high, such as around estuaries. It is common near oil fields and areas of seismic or volcanic activity.

Can geopathic stress be detected by machines?

The answer is yes and no. Some types can be readily detected and others are hard to detect.

There are two types of machines which can detect it. There are those which can detect its presence in people and those which can detect it on the ground. It may still be very difficult to detect even with very sophisticated equipment.

Devices which measure the electrical resistance of acupuncture points can detect its effects in people. These devices are known as electro-dermal screening devices.

Other methods may detect the presence of geopathic stress on the ground. Some of it may be detected by geo-magnetometers which can measure local magnetic fields; however they may not detect all types of geopathic stress.

The reason for this is that some geopathic stress consists of such extremely high frequency radiation that it is out of range of ordinary meters. The frequencies involved are 10 to the power of 23 Hertz and above. In other words, the number of cycles per second can be written as the number 10 followed by 23 zeroes. There exist in Germany prototype meters which can detect this frequency of radiation. However they are extremely expensive and at present are still experimental.

Dowsers and water diviners can also detect geopathic stress. This is a subjective method in as much as different dowsers may be tuned into different frequencies of radiation and so may come up with different results. However this can still prove an extremely useful method of detecting geopathic stress, especially in the absence of readily available and accurate meters.

How common is geopathic stress?

In my practice in Southern England I find that around 30% of patients are geopathically stressed. It seems to vary to some extent from one part of the country to another. It also varies from one country to another. For instance, it seems to be fairly common in Northern Australia where there is a lot of underground water which supplies artesian wells.

If geopathic stress is natural, why is it dangerous and why have we not become immune to it?

Although geopathic stress appears to have a natural origin in that it comes from the earth, a lot of it is nonetheless manmade.

According to the German scientist and expert on geopathic stress, Dr. Kohfink, there has been a huge increase in geopathic stress since the end of the second World War. The reason for this, he says, is the Nuclear Weapons Testing program and in particular, the underground nuclear tests.

He states that these have caused splits in the earth's crust that are 300 kms deep and that they allow extremely high frequency radiation from deep within the earth up to the surface. This radiation then goes 6,000 meters up above the earth's surface before dissipating.

As each nuclear test sends a shock wave 4 times around the whole earth, every country on earth has been affected by it.

Whether or not this explanation is correct, there is no doubt that there is a lot of geopathic stress around at the present time.

How do you treat geopathic stress?

Now we come to the good news. Geopathic stress is readily treatable. Essentially there are three ways of treating geopathic stress. These are:

1. To move out of the geopathic stress;
2. To block it and screen oneself;
3. To neutralize it.

As regards moving out of it, this does not usually mean moving house. Most people who are affected by geopathic stress are affected where they sleep as their bed is usually the only place in the house where they spend eight hours of every day without moving. Also the body's resistance to geopathic stress decreases markedly when we are asleep.

Therefore the primary and most effective way of dealing with geopathic stress is to move one's bed. This simple measure very often results in one moving out of the area of geopathic stress and it ceases to be a problem. The further the bed can be moved, the more likely it is that one gets out of the stressed area. However moving a bed by as little as two feet is sometimes sufficient to get out of the stressed area as it can be very localized. For some it is impossible to move their bed and in this case other methods need to be tried. These are worth doing anyway as a backup, even if it possible to move one's bed.

It is possible to block off geopathic stress by means of a layer of cork placed under the bed. A layer of cork tiles or bath mats, available from furniture stores, can be used. It is also possible to obtain large sheets of cork from specialist suppliers.

The scientific reason for this to work appears to depend on an observed association between geological fault lines and oak trees (which produce cork). The oak tree seems to have evolved its own defense against geopathic stress which is present in cork.

Last, there are ways of neutralizing geopathic stress. There are two main ways of doing this. One is by using devices or machines and the other is by means of dowsing.

The simplest device to neutralize that I know of is called 'The Charged Card' and is the size of a credit card. It can be carried in a pocket or kept within 2 feet of one's bed. It is inexpensive and effective.

Other devices which can be placed under the bed include Hartmann Spirals and Flat Dielectric Resonators which are made in the USA.

Another device is the Personal Energizer. It can be carried in a pocket or kept within 2 feet of one's bed. It is inexpensive and effective.

More costly are electronic machines which neutralize geopathic stress. These are plugged into the mains and then left on. They are capable of clearing an entire building of geopathic stress.

Finally there are dowsers who are able to clear it. Some will visit the house and clear the stress by driving metal stakes into the ground in order to divert the energy lines or by placing crystals to absorb it at key locations. There are also some dowsers who can clear a house by working on it at a distance using a floor plan of the house. Improbable as this seems, in my experience it can work. It may be explained scientifically by means of a physical principle known as Unified Quantum Field Theory.

This theory states that the control systems of living organisms exist at the level of the fifth dimension and therefore lie outside the four dimensional space-time continuum, which is all that we are ordinarily able to perceive of space and time. A deeper explanation of this theory lies beyond the scope of this article.

This is by no means a complete list of the ways of clearing geopathic stress. It represents one therapist's experience in treating it.

So what should I do if I think I may be geopathically stressed?

In order of importance, you should:
1. Move your bed if at all possible;
2. Place a layer of cork underneath it;
3. Get a Charged Card or similar device.

It is important to note that it may take six weeks for the effects of geopathic stress to clear. Also clearing geopathic stress on its own may not bring about a cure as you may need to take appropriate remedies as well.

If after doing all this you are no better after six weeks, you should consider:

1. Consulting a practitioner of German Biological Medicine;
2. Consider consulting a dowser;
3. Consider buying an electronic device to clear geopathic stress.

The most important thing to remember is that geopathic stress can in virtually every case be cleared.

FINDING THE TIME

Time for silence, time to listen, time for nature — how do we find it? Through mastering time. It begins by becoming proficient at time management.

If I filled a bottle completely full of beans, most would say it is full. But then I can still pour in a cup of salt that fills the spaces between the beans. Most would agree that the bottle is now completely full, but it is not so. I can still pour in half a cup of water. The use of time is like this; the big tasks that take up large amounts of time are the beans. But you can still fit well-planned little tasks into your day and these are the salt. Then little things can still be squeezed in with comfort – the water. Here are some suggestions:

• Scrutinize who brings you joy when you speak to them on the phone. Most call to avoid their own company, draining your energy and time. I change my phone number every few years; it's a minor inconvenience compared to unwanted phone calls. Keep the calls you wish to take brief.

• If you do like speaking with someone regularly, do a 'grains of salt' task by having earphones and a phone you can clip onto a belt. Mend a tear in a much loved teddy bear, a daughter's favorite blouse. Chop onions or peel potatoes for the whole week, to parboil and freeze in baggies. Mashed potatoes frozen in ice cube trays will thicken soups and sauces in a healthful way.

• The 'water in the bottle' tasks should have a little spot in rooms where you are likely to have a few minutes to spare; the kitchen while you wait for tea water to boil, the bathroom where you wait for the bath to fill. This is the time to write a quick note of thanks or encouragement. This can be the moment to remove the stain on a collar or sort a basket of socks or pre-make tomorrow's sandwiches.

• The large tasks require prioritizing. Do this daily. Uncompleted tasks are bumped to the next day's list so that nothing falls between the cracks.

> *"A life of grace produces refined awareness in your children. It is not the result of haphazard chaos but the culmination of a disciplined life lived with artistry and elegance."*
> —*Almine*

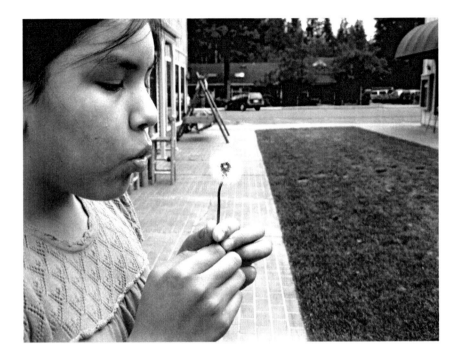

Teaching Children
to have Joy

"To live asleep is to think that life is duty. To awaken is to find that life is beauty. Many parents drive their children to acquire skill sets and achievements, forgetting to teach them how to be happy."

—Almine

"Use three physicians still: Doctor Quiet, next Doctor Merryman and Doctor Diet."

—Constantin the African

TEACHING CHILDREN TO HAVE JOY

Most parents cannot teach their children how to have joy because they do not know it themselves. Having lost the memory of what brings them joy during careworn or achievement-oriented years, they fill their own lives with incessant busyness. The role of parenting often is incorrectly seen as one of self-denial. If we abandon ourselves, how can we teach our children to be in touch with their own joy?

The child often comes between parents by demanding to sleep in their room or having a parent sleep in the child's room. The relationship between parents is the foundation of the home and they deserve a space and a time to foster it.

If a child is sent to daycare or preschool, it is preferable not to do so when he or she is two years old. Behavioral psychologists have determined this to be the critical age when a child learns to trust the stability of relationships with others. The realization that he will not be abandoned cannot be regained at a later age. Start your little one at one year old or at three, if possible.

The path of joy begins with the inner child. If we lose touch with that part of ourselves the pain of alienation sets in. This is the reason young teenagers feel so lost and have so much anguish. Trying to be grownup, they turn their back on their inner child's spontaneity and joy. Eventually this becomes a way of life, producing careworn, unhappy adults.

Nature provides a place where they can unselfconsciously be their integrated selves again. Lie with the child on your stomach next to a river, studying the story of the stones – what they tell about the ancient geological history of the area. Fry the fish they catch on an open fire. Try learning bird calls.

Joy comes from celebrating life and from random little surprises. Pick up their clothes, if you wish – greatness cannot be fostered in chaos. But insist on the tidiness of their minds. Help them with ruthlessness acknowledge that they are never victims of circumstances, but empowered beings masterfully creating the circumstances of their lives.

Be affectionate with touch and words and spontaneous acts of kindness. Turn back their sheets at night, stash lavender soaps in their drawers so their clothes smell nice, sort their clothes into color for easy mix and matching.

Each family member should know what little things and what large things make their hearts sing. Make lists you can keep adding to and put them up where they can be seen. Try budgeting time and money to fulfill these wishes as much as possible.

This also helps children see parents as more than agents to fulfill their needs, but as having needs themselves. Consideration in children must be taught by having them see through another's eyes. The nature of innocence is very similar to the sociological stage of tribalism – it is supremely self-centered.

A joyous day begins with grace. In the foyer all non-food items that must leave the house for school in the morning are laid out the night before. Lunches are laid out well before time to leave. If you have more than one child, there are piles of items. All the things you must remember for the office, for errands during the day are similarly laid out the night before. School clothes are laid out the night before as well.

Take a minute of time to have children cultivate the habit of envisioning how they want their day to unfold.

My daughter is very picky about whether and what she wants for breakfast. If she doesn't eat what I bring her for breakfast, I have a quick-to-fix backup snack to give her in the car. This seems to work and if it doesn't, I have just produced a mid-morning snack for myself.

It is a healthful habit to eat small, regular meals throughout the day. Of these, for many reasons including weight regulation, breakfast is the most important. Tempt children to eat, but do not force them, so that meals do not become a battleground. Have them sit and eat – any other posture can produce hiatal hernias over time. Don't discuss stressful subjects at mealtime.

> *"When you eat, just eat."*
>
> —*Zen proverb.*

Ways to Celebrate your Child

*"Love the body and allow this love to
penetrate every cell and heal you."*
—The Inner Door, Vol. I

CELEBRATING YOUR CHILD

1. Children of all ages, even infants, love massages of their neck and shoulders, backs, feet and hands. Almond oil works well for all ages. *Never* use mineral oil.

2. Go away for the weekend, unless you are breastfeeding an infant - but even then breast milk can be prepared ahead for a loving grandmother to give the child. Plan something unexpected – a fishing trip, a dinosaur dig, a Broadway show.

3. A surprise 'un-birthday' with a few wrapped presents and his or her favorite foods eaten by candlelight. A card can say, "Thank you for being my son/daughter."

4. Leave a note on their pillow with a treat to say, "To put a smile on your face, I'm doing your chores for the next two days. Enjoy!"

5. Make a scrapbook of his or her life with photos, certificates of achievement, mementos, the child's artwork. Leave it on his bed for him to enjoy in silence.

6. Tell your child you love him or her regularly. Tell them you want to be with them whenever they want you to. Ask them at times to help you garden, peel apples, knead dough, paint a room, wash the car. They may complain, but keep the activity short and ask them about their hopes and dreams and joys. What do they like most and least about school? What would they like to change in their lives?

7. Innovatively support their passions. They want to be a basketball player? Put up a net, take them to big games, rent videos. They want to be captain of their class? Help them organize their campaign. Make posters, produce pins.

Learning to Solve Problems with Skill and Finesse

"The barometer of the strength of a relationship is how well problems can jointly be solved. Rageful outbursts come from those who believe they have no other way to be heard."

—Almine

PROBLEM SOLVING – BASIC CONCEPTS

The basis of successful negotiations with another is the desire to learn, rather than to prove you are right. Children often want to be right at all costs because we praise them for winning rather than losing.

J.: I failed my state math exam.

M.: What did you learn?

J.: I don't like math.

M.: Let's go through and see exactly what the problem was. Failure can help us be better.

J.: Well, I didn't quite finish and I made a few careless mistakes.

M.: Did you run out of time?

J.: No, I didn't want to do it any more. Are you going to get me a tutor? I hate having tutors!!

M.: I have two questions; firstly, what's worse – to sit an extra 15 minutes and finish and check your math properly or to sit an hour a week for the next two months with a tutor? Secondly, a day without failure is often a day without growth. How did this failure make you better?

J.: Skipping doing the little things makes a lot more work in the end.

M.: Well done, Jaylene!

The fact that a child is sometimes right and a parent wrong is overlooked more often than not because of bias. Assume your child has much to teach you. Every soul is bedecked with jewels of insight. Listen objectively with your heart.

It is in fluidly and freely acknowledging when you are wrong that a child learns to be reasonable in adopting another's higher point of view. Teach by example that as long as you genuinely state your highest truth, being wrong has no shame attached to it. Tell him or her to diligently check that they are honest with themselves first, and others second. Give examples to younger children of what it means to lie to yourself.

It is a great disservice to your children to indulge any dysfunctionality. Dishonesty should have memorable consequences; a week of grounding or withholding of privileges. Stress the disrespect it is to you and how trust, once lost, cannot easily be regained. Tell smaller children a story such as *The Boy Who Cried Wolf.*

Make absolutely sure you are 100% honest with your children in word and deed. They sense when you are not or if there is dishonesty in the household. Even telling them there's a Santa Claus when there's not is enough to shake their confidence. Tell them you are both pretending there's a Santa so you can have a fun way of giving them presents.

Confrontation with hostility

• Teach your child to express confrontation this way:
> "When you do this (clearly state what is objectionable), I feel _____."

Tell them no matter how aggressive the opponent is, to keep bringing the interchange back to the statement above.

• The next step is to propose a possible solution. If the opponent does not agree, ask them for their alternative and see if any part of it is acceptable.

• Stress to your children that their feelings are always valid considerations.

• If tempers flare in older children, take the confrontation to written form. Ask them to think before they write, to avoid accusations, blame and phrases such as "you never' and "you always".

• Teach them that unsuccessful people in life say, "if only" and achievers say "next time".

• Tell them that for eagles to fly high they must be prepared to be rejected by the flocks of birds below them; that conformity is the death of greatness. True friends bring out our best and though they are hard to find, we attract them by being a friend. If we just continue to shine, others will eventually feel this gives them permission to shine also.

• Tell them you are their confidant and counselor and that together you can find ways to deal with bullies – never to be intimidated by them, but to let you know when they are encountered.

Understanding Conflict – A Parent's Guide

"Much of what we wish to teach our children we ourselves do not know. Throughout the generations dogma has replaced the skillful art of living impeccably. Let us learn together ..."

—Almine

HELPING PARENTS UNDERSTAND THE FOUR STAGES OF CONFLICT RESOLUTION

Stage 1

In the first stage of resolution we find common ground. Unless this is first identified we cannot properly determine which parts to resolve in Stage 2. Failure to determine what we have in common with the opposition robs us of the priceless gift of becoming more knowledgeable by learning new aspects and viewpoints of common ground. Too often opponents prematurely focus on the differences during this first stage instead of simply assimilating the commonalities so that these initial gifts of insight can be received.

Stage 2

In this stage of conflict resolution a closer scrutiny of what is the same and what is different must take place. Those unknown pieces must be examined in depth rather than taken at face value in order to extract common elements. It is necessary to examine these details in the context of the larger picture. Although we may have superficial differences, are we exploring a similar pattern? Are the core issues the same even though our method of dealing with them might be different? In this way the true differences to resolve are isolated from the similarities.

The last step is to creatively externalize them. Design a case scenario to objectively examine the issues as though they are happening to someone else. Reverse roles, honestly examining what it would be like to be in the other's shoes.

Stage 3

In conflict resolution this stage requires that we abandon our preoccupation with our own viewpoint and genuinely try to understand the opposing position. The need now arises to create a situation to test the validity of the opposing viewpoint; to see and understand it better by observing it in action. Where the stakes are high, the testing of the unknown can be done in multiple, smaller controlled settings.

Example: *Your teenager wants to date. You feel she's too young. She feels you're ruining her life because all her friends date. After completing the previous steps, one or two controlled situations could be tested wherein she is dropped off and picked up by you and has to call you if she changes locations. This option is opposed to one requiring an absolute yes or no with one party or the other feeling unheard. An informed conclusion can then be drawn as to what can be supported.*

Stage 4

In this stage we agree to disagree. The level of interaction is determined by what can be assimilated without being destructive to inner life or without being light- and growth-repressive. The key element of the success of this stage is to keep supporting the areas of common ground and the growth of all. Examples of the different degrees of interaction that could be allowed are:

• The in-laws don't like you, but they love your wife. Because they show their dislike when around you, you needn't be in their presence often but nevertheless can support your spouse being with them as she chooses. If their intent is destructive, such as to break up the marriage, this needs to be clearly identified and the interaction must then be very minimal or terminated, depending on the accompanying level of risk.

• If differences are only superficial but the common goals and philosophies are strong, we find we can live closely together or work together while honoring and supporting our diversity within our unity.

HOW PARENTS CAN LEARN TO DETERMINE WHETHER CONFLICT EXISTS

If we are walking a path of impeccability, it is imperative to suspend judgment when some seeming offense or disagreement occurs until we have obtained clarity. For example, some acquaintance hurts our feelings but we realized that words can mislead. We therefore ask,

"What did you mean when you said ....?" or "Why do you say such and such?" We do not ask in judgment, for no conclusion has been reached, but rather with an attitude of neutrality.

When we have ascertained the true meaning of what was said through feeling the intent behind the words and getting as much clarity as possible, we can proceed. Does it still bring our hackles up or create a knee-jerk reaction? If it does, we need to ask whether it is important enough to resolve with the other person or is it merely one of our 'buttons' that was pushed in order for us to examine some event in our own life that is waiting to yield its insights and power.

If it is important, however, it needs to be addressed. Here are some guidelines on how to decide what is important enough to merit confrontation:
• When there is hurtful intent or destructiveness.
• When it is injurious to the inner child, disrespectful to the sacred world of the inner sage or belittling to the inner nurturer.
• When it violates our privacy or our sacred space.
• When it violates our mutual agreement or trust or is dishonest in any way.
• When it belittles, suppresses our individuality or causes us to be less than we are.
• When it attempts to manipulate, control or dominate us.
• When it criticizes or accuses us.

If the incident fits one of the above scenarios, or a similar one, the following approach should be used:
• First of all, some basics should be agreed upon and perhaps even written.
• Within our relationships all feelings are valid – meaning we do not criticize another for feeling a certain way.
• All emotions should find a safe place for expression.
• Expressions such as "You always" or "You never" and "Why do you" should be prohibited when they are expressed as a disguised accusation rather than a simple question.
• Neither words nor emotions should be used to attack or manipulate.

- When someone is in the grip of uncontrollable rage, there should be preexisting coping mechanisms established. They are to wash their face and hands and/or engage in strenuous physical activity to organize their thoughts before expressing them.
- Writing letters that are not dispatched is another productive form of communication when there are rage issues.

Feelings must be expressed and a solution proposed by the confronting person. This may have to be done a few times before achieving results. "When you do this, I feel this. Is it possible that in future we can try such and such?"

The appropriate way for the other person to respond is to first make sure they understand. "Are you saying that …?" if they acknowledge that a change in behavior is appropriate it is advisable to create a backup plan since deep-seated habits are hard to break.

Can we have a secret hand gesture or phrase to remind you when old habits creep in?" or "Could I pull you aside to remind you of that?"

If instead the other person starts venting, sit absolutely still and let it run its course until it is spent. Then repeat what you said, always bringing the conversation back to the relevant point. If this does not work, write it out and request a written response within a few days. If the conflict persists, there are only three choices remaining:

1. **Evaluate** whether what you have in common contributes sufficiently to your life for you to continue to put up with the differences. If the differences are more significant, either sever the relationship or be prepared for ongoing discomfort.

2. **Flow** around the obstacles because the relationship has been determined to be worth saving. Be creative. He embarrasses you in public? Create a private world for your interaction and make as many public appearances as possible alone. It is never a good idea to force round pegs into square holes.

3. **Change** your attitude. Even if you do the damage control suggested in #2 there are still going to be odd times when the offensive behavior will happen. Lift yourself above the situation like the eagle that flies above the earth. Envision yourself sitting in an insulating

bubble of pinkish purple light, holding your inner child and talking to it during the occurrence.

It is never to the benefit of indwelling life to accept the unacceptable. It is also eroding to have many 'little' occurrences happening day in and day out. How diligently is the person working on improving him or herself? All these factors must be taken into consideration in coming to a final conclusion. Another helpful tool is to picture enduring this behavior for the next ten years and weighing it against the positive aspects of the relationship.

Being a Peacemaker

"Peace at the cost of truth cannot be long lasting. Truth must surface, for all of the cosmos conspires to right a wrong."

—*Almine*

ACKNOWLEDGING TRUTH – THE FIRST STEP IN PEACEMAKING

Light-promoters frequently make the mistake of seeing physical concerns through the rose-colored glasses of a spiritual vantage point and then treating them as though they are in fact spiritual rather than physical. Some examples of this would be:

• Bill loves his brother Sam but his childhood experiences have made him inclined to find security in wealth. Through conniving manipulation, Bill cheats Sam out of his share of their inheritance. Because Sam can see how Bill has suffered and how much money means to him and because he also knows that deep down Bill loves him, he lets him get away with it.

Conclusion: Sam believes himself to be acting magnanimously but in fact he is injuring Bill. Bill can now continue to see his theft as cleverness, allowing him to create karma that will call forth similar circumstances on his own head. If he doesn't see clearly when he reaps that karma, it will have to happen again and again. Sam has foregone the opportunity to lovingly and firmly let Bill know that his conduct is unfair and unacceptable.

• Mary's eldest daughter seems to be floundering in every area of her life and Mary feels guilt because she believes she is partly responsible for not having been a better parent during a time when she was floundering herself. She keeps saving her daughter and as a result, finds she has to do without in order to manage her budget.

Conclusion: Seeing the reason for someone's shortcomings doesn't excuse them. We may have compassionate understanding for the cause of their behavior, but to indulge the behavior keeps that person locked into that position. Compensating for lack in someone else's perception robs them of the opportunity to grow. When we keep someone from growing just to ease our guilt, we are acting selfishly.

If we serve the growth of all concerned, we will not view our role as peacemaker as one of covering someone's folly. To promote peace means to enhance growth as effortlessly as possible and sometimes it means exposing someone's flawed viewpoint. It would also mean

helping someone ask the type of questions that could set them free from the treadmill of lack of perception. An example of this could be:
• There are three friends, Jan, Sue and Beth. Sue and Beth get into a disagreement and try to solve it through letters to each other. Sue sends all letters first to Jane to 'check over', asking whether they sound too adversarial and posing various other questions that skirt the main issue; that she is broaching a verbal agreement upon which Beth has relied and acted for many months. Jane loves both her friends and wants to make peace. She therefore focuses on helping Sue write as nicely as possible, attempting to answer the irrelevant questions that divert focus from what is really going on.

She scrupulously tries to avoid giving advice, not pointing out that the questions don't really lead to the discovery of the core disagreement or problem, but actually prolong it. As Sue asks more and more friends to advise her and all give a neutral response or advice positive to her position (not knowing both viewpoints), she deviates further and further from the core question: "Did I have a verbal agreement my friend depended on and am I going back on my word?" The mirrors around her have given no hint of any flaws in her reasoning and she is therefore becoming more convinced by the moment that her actions are justified.

If, on the other hand, Jan realizes that by playing this avoidance game with Sue she is not being a friend to either Sue or Beth, she may ask instead, "Where is the area of blindness in this matter?" She may then, after gathering the facts from both sides, find the core of the disagreement. When this is pointed out with love to one friend or another, the disagreement at least has a chance to be healed sooner rather than later.

In an attempt to avoid taking sides, or in a misguided effort to focus on the positive (which helps only if one is also prepared to point out the flaws in perception), peacemakers tend to complicate things. Every challenge has a core mystery or blind spot. No matter how much clearing has to be done, it must be accomplished for all involved to grow.

As peacemakers our task is to reveal the root of the conflict; to serve only indwelling life rather than the mirrors of illusion. Mirrors entrap – the truth sets us free.

Leadership through Authentic Living

"One who lives authentically from the heart is self-referring for approval. To such a one, leadership as a means of persuading others is meaningless. He or she simply shines like the brightest star in the sky and others, seeing such a light, are inspired to find their own as well."

—*Almine*

CONCEPTS OF LEADERSHIP TO INSTILL IN OUR CHILDREN

- We are stewards of our Earth, our bodies and our environment. We pick up trash on the ground, we self-nurture our bodies, watching with care what we feed them. We take care of our possessions. We mend and fix what we can so that we do not carelessly add to the trash heaps of the Earth. We service our cars and appliances regularly. We do not allow others to destroy our property or defile our home.
- We live our highest truth, no matter whether others approve or not. In being home for ourselves we cease to need. In ceasing to need, we are no longer able to be controlled by the games of others.
- We are content alone, with a good book if we choose. When we choose to be with another it is not because we feel we must, but because they enhance our lives. When that is no longer the case we gracefully walk the other way, fluid as the river and free as the wind. Tell your child that many grownups are unhappy because they are afraid to be alone.
- Give the children many decisions to make: "Do you want to play with your puzzle or are you going to put on an apron and stand on a chair to help me wash the dishes?" The more you give them to decide for themselves, the more robust their leadership abilities will become.
- The great and exceptional people of the world have been those who have found their way out of societal conformity. Vigorously guard against allowing society's value systems into your home. Avoiding programmed status symbols and societal dictates are compelling reasons why our home has no television. My daughter is an innocent 11 year old, not an 11year old behaving like a 14 year old. I have invited her to discuss freely with me all sexual questions. I feel content that I am the source of her information, not the television.
- One of the largest engineering firms in the US has encountered a dilemma; their young, computer-raised engineers cannot talk to

the older generation of engineers. One of the clear deficiencies in those who get all their information form computers is the inability to think abstractly. Not having learned through hands-on experience, they cannot envision some concepts until they see them in two-dimensional diagrams. As a parent you must decide for yourself, but I am in no hurry for Jaylene to have a computer. What she learns at school will have to suffice for now.

AUTHENTIC ACHIEVEMENT

In order to assess your child's abilities, there is something vital that must be considered. Is he a horizontal or vertical thinker? Parents need to familiarize themselves with these proclivities.

Stalkers versus Dreamers
(Excerpt from *Journey to the Heart of God*)

Humanity consists of both right-and left-brained individuals. We shall call the right brained ones Dreamers and the left brained ones Stalkers. Those approaching life through the left brain, the Stalkers, have what is called a vertical approach to life. The right brained Dreamers approach life horizontally.

The Stalkers access more of the vertical mental waves of awareness and the Dreamers the horizontal waves. Stalkers access the known deeply and analytically, like a flashlight shining a small, bright, clearly defined beam of light onto a wall. Dreamers access more of the unknown, like a wide circle of diffused light. Stalkers can juggle twelve balls in the external world for every one the Dreamers can. But Dreamers will pick up many times more non-cognitive information.

The way Dreamers access the world has been very much misunderstood. The educational system is designed around the way Stalkers think. As it is, Stalkers can grasp external information at the rate of thirty-four units to every twenty-one units the Dreamers can. The Dreamers have consequently traditionally been underestimated as under-achievers.

Stalkers in Relationships

• In personal relationships Dreamers find Stalkers cold and calculating at times. They are less inclined to make small talk and think they're helping by analyzing their partners or the situation.

• Stalkers often fire facts at coworkers or employees in a way that reminds one of a machine gun. They may pause for breath just long enough to ask whether there are any questions, since they may be seeing a dazed expression on the face of Dreamer listeners. However, the Dreamers can't assimilate such a deluge of information, get lost early in the conversation and don't even know at this point what the questions are. Instructions to your Dreamer child may have the same response.

• Stalkers feel unheard because after 'carefully explaining' in great detail, it's clear that nobody seems to do as instructed. (No one understood.)

• Stalkers may ask Dreamers a question (since they seldom make small talk because they find it abstract or profound) and get unclear or evasive answers. Again, they feel unheard and do not understand that Dreamers process a question by internalizing it; feeling it in their heart. Only then will they think it over. It could take days.

• Stalkers feel particularly unheard when voicing their feelings. A typical conversation between a Stalker husband and Dreamer wife might go as follows:

> *The husband comes home from work and complains that the lunch she makes him every day is giving him heartburn. She is washing the dishes, hardly looks up and says, "That's nice, dear. By the way, the upstairs toilet is plugged. Would you fix it?" He thinks she doesn't care, but what she has really said is that it's not the lunch; his 'plumbing' is backed up. She doesn't know herself what her words mean. She just accesses it. He's supposed to analyze it.*

Dreamers in relationships

• Dreamers feel unheard by Stalkers. The Stalkers find Dreamers' questions to be out of place, not on track or not to the point. They are therefore often dismissed as not contributing or being irrelevant.

• When Dreamers express their feelings they are often very emotional and appear to the frustrated Stalker to be irrational or illogical. When a Stalker husband tries to create order from his Dreamer wife's 'ramblings', she feels he is not honoring the process of her feelings.

There are great gifts Stalkers and Dreamers can give each other. The Dreamers have a knack for improving the quality of the journey through life. They may take longer to reach the goal, but the end product is often more creative. They provide a lot of energy to Stalkers through their association.

Stalkers are goal-minded and bring organization to the Dreamer's life. They are good at running daily life and creating order out of chaos, something that appeals to Dreamers who frequently have difficulty keeping the physical aspects of their lives in order.

Until Dreamers and Stalkers see how to utilize the respective gifts each mindset brings to a relationship, the friction between them will be ongoing. Many of us still look for uniformity in our relationships, which brings stagnation rather than growth. The goal of having unity within diversity promotes the most growth but requires understanding, patience and the tolerance necessary to support each other's differences.

How Stalkers and Dreamers can bridge the communication gap
If the two different camps want to communicate, they will have to learn each other's skill sets.

Tools for Dreamers
• Dreamers can be seen as slow since, as previously discussed, their ratio of assimilating new information is twenty-one to thirty-four in respect to Stalkers. It will assist them to cultivate the tool of speed-reading. Colleges offer classes in this.
• Dreamers get overwhelmed when bombarded by information. They either need to take a proper shorthand course or develop their own shorthand system.

• Dreamers hold long term memory patterns well but not short term memory. They have to cultivate better short term memory by practicing with pieces of information they can afford to fail with. Read a phone number once, dial the whole number; do the same with an address. When typing something on the computer, try to type longer and longer pieces without looking at notes.

• When given complex instructions, use shorthand. Then take time to digest and sort out what has been said. See if there are any gaps in the information and then formulate concise but comprehensive questions to obtain the missing pieces; do not be afraid to ask.

• Remember that Stalkers will hold you accountable for every word you say.

Tools for Stalkers

• Stalkers should identify the Dreamers in their environment and slow down the instructions or conversation by using metaphors, examples, stories and humor. When Stalkers are speaking too fast, Dreamers cannot ask questions since they do not even know what to ask.

• Stalkers must remember that Dreamers are generally far more intelligent than they are perceived to be, but the system has not allowed them to shine. Remember too that most people are Dreamers.

• Stalkers have often become impatient, confrontational, blaming or controlling with Dreamers and when this happens Dreamers tend to shut down.

• Stalkers will isolate themselves from others unless they loosen their expectations. By being over-focused on results they can alienate the rest of the team.

• Stalkers need to have what to them seems like 'meaningless social interaction' in order to get Dreamers to relax around them so the Stalkers can be heard. If the Stalker has a Dreamer boss, social coworkers may be promoted over him because of the value Dreamers place on the quality of the journey.

• Stalkers must remember that most Dreamers say things they don't mean when emotional. They should at least try and listen behind the words to their intent, using the heart rather than the head. Ask a few questions when the emotions are spent (too many will make Dreamers feel interrogated). Developing listening skills is the number one skill for Stalkers to cultivate in trying to bridge the gap.

Developing
Omni-sensory Perception

*"It is in our children that the future evolution-
ary leaps of man are visible. We assist n the
metamorphosis of man by fostering them."*

—*Almine*

NURTURING YOUR CHILD'S OMNI-SENSORY PERCEPTION

"Our children come, trailing clouds of glory from afar ..."
—William Wordsworth

Extrasensory perception

The vast majority of life around us is not visible to most people. Cats can see the hidden realms as can some dogs.[16] The extraordinary children being born can, too – that is, until most parents program this ability out of them. This is done in the following ways:

• By negating, disbelieving or denying children's experiences either because we don't believe there are realities beyond what we can see or because we think it is part of their fantasy world.

• By signaling or feeling fear of the unknown and not trusting the benevolence of the hidden realms. Fear is often present if the child's abilities are seen as mental instability or if they set them apart from others in a way that will ostracize them from their peers. Do we really want the extraordinary to be suppressed simply in order to be acceptable to the mediocrity of the masses?

Teach your child early that they have a special gift others do not – not even yourself; that they have 'special eyes and ears'. Tell them to share their experiences with you – you would love to know what you are missing. Then listen, even if it sounds farfetched. Look at the inter-dimensional photos on www.interdimensionalphotos.com to see just how amazing the hidden realms really are. Your child may lack the vocabulary necessary to explain his experiences. If so, have him draw it.

Explain how many in history, like Galileo, have been misunderstood by their peers. Tell you child to share his or her gifts only at home where they are welcomed and enjoyed.

• Your child may have night terrors by seeing things in the bedroom. It is easier to see inter-dimensionally in the dark or semi-

---

16   See www.interdimensionalphotos.com.

dark. Instead of telling the child that what they see is not real, hold them in a comforting embrace and have them:

    a) describe the being to you;

    b) ask the being what it wants and then ask your child to tell you (assuming the child is clairaudient as well as clairvoyant). If he or she does not hear anything, ask the child to sit very still and feel what the being wants.

• By your trying to provide answers for your child, even though this may be an area about which you know nothing. It is the officious arrogance of man to think that his established religions, belief systems and pat answers can explain anything about the ever-new unfolding wonders of the universe. It is the beginning of greatness to acknowledge that we know nothing. It is a valuable gift to a child when a parent can demonstrate through example that there is nothing to know and everything to explore.

• Parental protectiveness often blinds us to the fact that our child is masterfully manifesting his or her own life's circumstances. By all means safeguard your child from potentially hazardous events. It is unlikely that the hidden realms will present these, but if your child has strong feelings that a being is hostile, you may chase it way with strong commands. Remember that some beings, like tree spirits, look very outlandish but are actually benign.

> *There are more things in heaven and earth, Horatio,*
> *Than are dreamt of in your philosophy.*
>   —Wm. Shakespeare, Hamlet, *Act I*

Omni-sensory perception

Special capacity children have been called 'Indigo' children, 'Crystal' children and many other names[17]. Whatever they are called, it is clear that their senses have greater capacities than the norm. They may 'hear' telepathically the tones or songs emitted by flowers, stars, etc. Their sensory input may be overwhelming as it is, but add to that the blaring television or noise at school and they may become dis-

---

17 See www.awakeningstarseeds.com/indigocrystal.htm.

sociative in order to cope. They then run the risk of being branded with Attention Deficit Disorder. They need lots of quiet time, alone time and time for integration (coming home from school or an activity). Talk to them about what they hear and see so that their special gift does not isolate them.

Fostering omni-sensory perception

• Encourage your children to do experimental exercises such as trying to taste the sound of music or hearing the sound of colors.
• Have they try to hear with the whole body or to see through their skin.
Note: There have been a number of studies testing and documenting the ability of individuals to cross-perceive sensory input. The most extensive are probably the experiments conducted by Russian scientists during the cold war as part of their programs in enhanced espionage techniques. Helen Keller was also reputed to be able to sense some sound and color vibrations through her skin.

Dealing with the gift of empathy

One of my children was so empathic that he could not stand to walk past the children's shoes at school; the pain of their lives spoke too clearly to him and he felt it as his own. A problem often experienced by empaths is their inability to distinguish whether the feelings involved are his own or those of others.

It is not always easy to spot the empathic qualities of a child. He or she may just seem to be moody. Carefully observe whether the moods of others in your child's environment are affecting him. If so, ask him to see how it makes him feel when someone in his environment is sad, angry or happy.

Once you have jointly established that your child is taking on the feelings of others, explain how this can cause him or her to be like a puppet on a string. If someone pulls his 'sad string', your child will respond to that emotion. Make it clear how important it is to live free from others' strings that can determine how we should feel.

How to cope with empathic feelings
• Tell your child to see if what he is feeling belongs to him or to someone else.
• Have him ask, "If the other person didn't feel this way, would I?"
• Once he knows he is feeling someone else's pain, etc., tell him to see it coming from that person – perhaps like a colored breeze. Anger could be red, sadness could be blue. Tell him to let the breeze go right through him and to make sure it does not stick.
• He or she could use a breathing technique – breathing in the other's emotion and then blowing it out. If there is physical distress in the body, pretend there is a mouth in that area and blow the tightness or discomfort out.

Life at School for a Sensitive Child

"The more you provide heaven on Earth at home, the more stark the contrast when the child goes to school. Yet the solace of a loving, cherishing environment to come home to is a source of great strength in the face of the often brutal atmosphere of school."

—*Almine*

CULTIVATING INDIVIDUALITY IN THE FACE OF PEER PRESSURE

You nurture the individuality and exceptional qualities in your child by providing him or her with an exceptional life. Confidence to boldly and authentically express comes from exceptional experiences. It is quite fine to be different, if by 'different' it means a richer, fuller, more exciting life; a life peers would love to be a part of.

Creating such a life for you and your child requires extra effort and planning – and, if you wish – budgeting of money and time.

Low budget activities

• A trip to the local pound or pet store to pet the puppies and kittens. I have an arrangement with the local pet store for Jaylene to be their 'official puppy petter'. I take my work, sit in the car while she gives love and affection to the little animals. Her friends love to join us.

• Camping trips with a purpose:
  ○ White water rafting;
  ○ Fossil gathering;
  ○ Looking for hidden treasure (that you hid for them);
  ○ Bird watching;
  ○ Learning about rocks;
  ○ Finding remnants of history.

• Slumber parties that have (under supervision) outrageous activities such as:
  ○ A movie marathon that lasts all night;
  ○ A midnight swim and picnic breakfast;
  ○ A candlelight dinner at midnight.

• Take family car trips to no destination to see where you end up. Or plan trips to hot springs or observatories. Take lots of provisions.

• We go to thrift stores, dollar stores, junk shops where children can do their own shopping with their own money. They buy outrageous glitter, high-heeled shoes and other things that make them feel special and abundant.

- We find any excuse to have a party:
  - o Making ice cream;
  - o Making apple cider;
  - o Decorating cookies;
  - o Silly hat tea parties;
  - o Watching meteor showers;
  - o Calling 'bigfoot' parties;
  - o Game parties with prizes.

More expensive outings

- Cross country train trips
- Visits to national parks
- Grand hotel visits
- Seeing scenic wonders by car
- Boat cruises
- Visiting foreign countries
- Opera and ballet performances
- Large museums of all types

Enriching the home life

- Turn off all the lights for one night, light candles and a fire and tell stories.
- Sit around a bonfire and share:
  - o Most embarrassing stories
  - o Silly things we did when we were small
  - o Things I like most about me
  - o And more …
- Roast supper foods on an open fire.
- Have dinner outside on a picnic blanket.
- Have messy finger painting art projects on big plastic sheets.
- Be innovative with menus and dinner presentations.
- Put surprises in their lunch boxes and little packages on their pillows.

- Teach them skills like making jam from fruit they pick.
- Watch the sunset together and teach them about the stars.
- Jaylene loves riding around town at night, watching the lights. This is even better at Christmas as we sing our favorite songs.
- Have them choose foods for supper occasionally.
- Cuddle with them, praise them and tell them you love them regularly.

Confidence through being taken seriously

Jaylene's artwork is on my blog, my online institute courses and framed upon my mantle where it is placed along side expensive artwork. At times I 'commission' art from her and use it in a book. I tell her she is very helpful in my work. She knows I am a single mother and that I work joyfully to provide for us. It means a lot to her that she can help.

She has modeled for the Shrihat Satva Yoga manual, earning money for her Christmas shopping. She has a little folder I made her called *The Modeling Portfolio of Jaylene*. She has earned blue ribbons at the fair for her canning (proudly displayed on a kitchen shelf), cooking, dried flower arrangements (we dry them ourselves) and art. I have framed these for her.

I honor her achievements and celebrate her life. At times I have had to buy her clothes at second-hand stores, but she has always been beautifully dressed with care. I take her seriously.

Solving school problems

We treat all Jaylene's teachers like family, with gratitude and respect. We recognize that theirs is often a thankless job and honor them with flowers and other gifts on Mother's Day, Valentine's Day, Christmas, etc. They in turn treat Jaylene respectfully, providing a place for her to go if she is in distress. I am there to help them if they need me and they are there for my daughter. It is a treasured relationship and teaches Jaylene gratitude.

We try to preempt problems. We have mapped out a course of action to take before something like bullying or menacing occurs.

We have discussed what to do when menstruation occurs, when she needs to contact me in case she feels unwell, and so on. We even look at what could provoke the animosity of others. In this way she is prepared and less likely to be taken by surprise.

Tutors

It is a bad habit to accept failure as the norm. If a child has a problem with a specific subject at school, either set aside time each week to tutor them yourself or have someone qualified tutor them for you. It is money well spent when failure is turned into success. At times teachers themselves are happy to spend an hour or so after school to help.

Having friends

Teach your children that when you are happy to be your own best friend (something they learn at home with solo-play) it is not essential to have friends. From a parent's concerned attitude, a friendless child can feel like a failure. Prepare them for this possibility by:
• Discussing alternative activities if they are alone at recess (a good book, for instance).
• Having them practice with you on how to initiate conversation with a prospective new friend.
• Finding out whether there are peers they would like to have you invite over.
• Giving the message clearly that solitude is preferable to having the 'wrong' friend.

The Learning Experience - from Infancy to Adulthood

"Education is the navigation of the mind-made maze of man that acquaints us with its stale information. Stimulated learning is the remembering of the all-knowingness of the self – the seat of effortless genius."

—*Almine*

METHODS TO STIMULATE LEARNING

Stimulating Learning in Infancy

Within the womb the infant floated effortlessly in the amniotic fluid, safe, warm and secure within his mother's heartbeat. From this haven, birth must seem unimaginably traumatic. To lessen the shock of entering the separation consciousness of the wide world, Maria Montessori, founder of the Montessori school and learning program, wrote:

> *"The child must remain as much as possible in the first few days in contact with his mother. There must not be too much contrast as regards to warmth, light and noise with his conditions before birth ...*
>
> *We may say that the child has merely changed his position in regard to her: he is now outside her body instead of inside. But everything else remains the same and communication between them still exists."*

A quiet period of rest for both the mother and child allows them to fully recover from the birth experience.

Studies in orphanages in Iran indicate that early stimulation and interaction of infants and toddlers enhances intelligence. Maria Montessori writes:

> *"The first lesson we must learn is that the tiny child's absorbent mind finds all its nutrients in its surroundings. It builds itself up from what it takes in. especially at the beginning of life we must, therefore, make the environment as interesting and attractive as we can."*

There should be many pictures on the walls, moving mobile toys above the crib and a sloping support behind the baby's back to enable him to see his environment, not just a blank ceiling.

Native Americans and Africans have the infant either on the Mother's back where he can look out at the world or – in the case of Native Americans – hanging vertically from a tree, safely wrapped and swaddled in a 'papoose'. This stimulates the baby's curiosity about his world.

The voice and face of the mother evokes deep feelings in the infant, stimulating depth in its emotional development. Talk to your baby; sing and croon. Teach baby to consciously grasp by placing your finger in his tiny hand and providing lots of soft, attractive, light weight rattles and stuffed animals for him to hold.

Experts believe that keeping an infant on its back prevents crib deaths. But place baby on his or her tummy, un-swaddled, on a blanket on the floor for at least half an hour a day so he can learn to hold up the head and explore different ways of moving.

Stimulating Learning in Small Children

In her book, *Montessori Insights for Parents of Young Children*, Aline Wolf writes about creating a safe haven in our homes for exploring toddlers. She advocates anticipating what the toddler would want to explore by going into each room and sitting on the floor at the child's level. Remove possibly injurious objects. Cover electrical outlets and protect stairways, table coverings that could be pulled down and floor lamps that could be knocked over.

Vacuum or sweep the floor area every day to eliminate small objects your infant could choke on. Let people remove their shoes before coming into the home and keep the flooring as germ-free as possible.

Aline Wolf writes:

"Be careful not to let concern for your home environment or your own activities restrict your toddler from the free exercise that optimizes his physical and mental development."

This is the crucial age for building confidence. Your child must learn that it is safe to enthusiastically reach for his world.

Stimulating Learning in Early Childhood

Read to your children as a daily routine. Introduce them to the wealth of stimulating books and story hours at your public library.

Montessori is a highly recommended educational program that did wonders for Jaylene's self-confidence in a very loving, nurturing, home-away-from-home atmosphere. Concentration is sometimes more difficult for exceptional children because of their expanded awareness. Montessori activities are specifically designed to lengthen concentration and attention spans.

> "Respect for each child's attention is very evident throughout the room as a Montessori teacher rarely interrupts a child who is focused on her work."
> —*Aline Wolf*

Older Children and Television

As children become older, all too often the primary educator becomes television. Take control of this runaway situation as early as possible, but at any age if you must. Establish firm rules if the home must have a television. In all 11 years of Jaylene's life, we have never had television reception in our home. We use televisions only for well-chosen videos.

Television rules
- No television viewing for toddlers.
- No use of television as a babysitting tool.
- No television when the day begins, before school.
- No television should be on when no one is watching.
- Limit television watching to an hour or hour-and-a-half per day.
- Prerecord good programs and eliminate the brainwashing of advertisements.
- Monitor what they are watching to prevent pollution of your child's mind.

Stimulating Learning in Older Children and Teenagers
Parental guidance
1. Involve yourself in what they are studying at school, enlisting the cooperation of your child's teacher. Do extra-credit projects

with them. Take them on field trips that will make the subject matter come alive.

2. Allocate much time for your children. Bearing children and providing for their physical needs only is not parenting; it is procreating. To raise an exceptional child requires dedicated parental skills.

3. The use of negative adjectives and name calling must *never* be a part of raising your exceptional child. A child becomes what you label them. It may be a naughty action to put gum in his sister's hair, but always keep the message consistent. He is a wonderful and exceptional child who has made a non-life-enhancing choice. A good child like yours makes life better. Convey to him that to make life worse is not in keeping with his high qualities.

The same approach will have to be used when you say 'no' to what other parents in their indifference allow. The music and filth coming through MTV is at times shockingly obscene. You can't put filth in and expect impeccability to come forth in your child's actions.

> "The utmost care in selective sensory input needs to be taken. Once smut has been seen or heard, it cannot be unseen or unheard. High mindedness and character are not grown in mud."
>
> —Almine

BODY-MIND DEVELOPMENT AND NATURAL WELLNESS IN YOUTH

Rory C. Mullin, MSc

Children In Motion

The growth and development from childhood to adulthood transpires through the interaction of many different variables. To be born into this world and navigate through its opportunities and barriers is a unique and adventurous process. The path to achieving an existence of health, happiness and longevity is initiated at conception and continues until physical death, requiring many tools and strategies to survive, manage and excel at any given time. There are levels of evolution through which an individual child grows, learns and progresses to effectively live as an adult.

A child need not be controlled, but merely nurtured and equally guided to provide protection and direction for their unfolding life. In essence, the growing child needs love, support, feeding and protection from harm. Physical movement is the laid foundation for complete integration of body-mind-spirit. Physical movement of a child displays a need for interface with a variety of types and styles for health of the whole person.

"The disablement of the body delivers its impression to the mind. Disablement of the mind delivers to impression to the body." (PC)

The body-mind is an intricate and inseparable entity. The body wears the mind. Thus the physical body reflects the health and current representation of the mind and its accumulated experiences. This is an important consideration, when at present a high number of youth exist with obesity issues, diabetes, soft tissue trauma, mental-emotional disorders and who are utilizing synthetic food supplements and pharmacological medication. You may want to investigate or observe for yourself the level of health and excellence displayed by the youth of today, who are the adults of future.

In every child or maturing adult, there exist certain stages of progressive development that allow human nature to naturally unfold in a process of continued evolution. The survival and evolution of the human being is dependent on the triad of body, mind and spirit integration. While often spoken of separately as segregated entities, the three exist in union. For example:

> *Car frame ~ body (structure)*
> *Engine ~ mind (emotions)*   *Whole Health*
> *Gasoline ~ spirit (life force)*

For whole health, a person requires balance and integration of all three.

The body and mind are describable in division and do have distinct functions, but interact synergistically as one. This inseparable connection has been observed in science, metaphysics and esoteric literature.

Candice Pert (*Molecules of Emotion*) states:

> *"Neuropeptides and their receptors are keys to understanding how mind and body are interconnected, and how emotions can be manifested throughout the body. Indeed, the more we know about neuropeptides, the harder it is to think in traditional terms of a mind and a body. It makes more and more sense to speak a single integrated entity, a 'body-mind'."* (p.WPM)

Body-mind integration and mutually inclusive development, relate to the quality of growth and development a child moves through. (LH.WBM) This integration is holism, an approach in creating whole health. Body-mind connection is not dualistic in nature and functions as an integrated operating unit, with no set lines of demarcation.

Upon conception the child starts its path of evolutionary growth. The infant child is in constant motion, with each movement a response to an internal sensation or external environment. Sandow stated: *"Life is movement. Movement – self-movement – is life.*

The fundamental phenomenon of all organic life is change of form (or movement)." (p.130 - *Life is Motion* – 1929)

Parental Suggestion

It is crucial that at the onset of your child's life, parental awareness exists of the importance of motor development through motion. Current societal values emphasize learning without establishing the body-mind connection in its entirety. Various critical development stages exist during childhood that, when missed through depriving them of physical expression cannot be retrieved. Parental education about the vital role of exercise throughout the child's life is crucial.

Infant Development

There are stages of progressive development for infant growth that have been observed and studied. Moving effectively through these stages is essential and leads to enduring health to follow. This crucial period, during the early months is the foundation for activating the sensory-motion system (feel-move), followed by other functional tissues and systems. Infants initially learn by 'moving to feel,' then later 'feeling to move.' So the initial movements are its initial sense. This is critical with the movement patterns being progressively sequenced to allow for an optional outgrowth, and later serve as a foundational platform for learning and complex movements.

"Infants are born as motor-sensory beings because the motor nerves to the extremities are as yet un-myelinated[18]; they learn to sense, to feel, through the process of learning to move. The world becomes a source of feedback. Via movement, infants learn to feel themselves. As they learn to feel themselves, they learn how to feel and navigate the environment(s) they are in." (PC) (CP2)

---

18 Myelinate- to cover or coat. A medical term in neurophysiology referring to a process in which the neural sheath develops a fatty deposit surrounding the nerve axon- to protect and enhance neural conductivity.

This sensory-motor stage aids the infant in differentiating front/ back, left side/right side, upper/lower body. These subtle developments create greater perception and awareness for greater growth. There are numerous small details that integrate form and function.

Avoid paralysis by analysis. Don't allow the mind (thoughts and ideas) to limit or restrict potential. Greater perception is complementary to power essence. Increased awareness and perception lead to increase in power potential. Perception is how one relates to what we are sensing; it is about relationship to self, other, environment.

"One of the things that I think is essential with sensing, is that we reach a point where we become conscious and then we let it go, so that the sensing itself is not a motivation, that our motivation is action based on perception." (BBC)

Infant developmental deficiencies may show up at various ages if growth is incomplete or inadequate to meet the desired demands of completing a task. Deficiencies may be subtle and show up as poor posture, inefficient gait, poor movement skills, chronic soft tissue dysfunction, visceral pathology, mental emotional balance and disharmony of body-mind.

As an adult we often come to a point where we want to learn more about our self so we may be better able to navigate through life. We may get caught up in externalizing our focus/energy, rather than internalizing. This is a body-mind reflection and balancing. Increased knowledge of self allows for increased understanding and improved awareness. With infants and youth as a whole, internal and external environments are all new experiences, adventures and opportunities to learn and grow.

It is through our senses that we receive information from our internal environment (self) and the external (outer world). Through our five senses (smell, taste, hear, sight, touch) and the functions of our nervous system, we filter numerous pieces of information to elicit a response or non-response. Touch, feel, taste, sense and movement are the first of the senses to develop, and thus set up or establish a baseline for (future) perception through taste, smell, hearing and vision. Mouth and hand to mouth is of the first motor command. Information gives something meaning. It is a gathering, validating, observing, evaluating and judging of what is perceived to them individuality (safe/unsafe, love/pain).

Breathing is an internal movement type and affects body movements and mental states. It is breath which initiates our first perceived independence and separation from other and our source of freedom and health. Breathing, right from the first 'breath of life,' is organized in patterns, which are influenced by emotional stimuli (or holding patterns) and evoke emotional responses. When uninhibited, each pattern fully develops and automatically transitions into succeeding patterns of a process of cumulative complexity.

"Aligning inner cellular awareness and movement with outer awareness and movement through space within the context of the development process can facilitate the evolution of our consciousness and alleviate body-mind problems at their root level." (p.6 BBC-S, F&A) Sense, Feeling & Action 8-92 articles

It may seem minimal and not of that much immediate importance, but these subtle and refined details in a child's upbringing set the foundation on which life may be experienced and managed in an effective manner. Growth and development do not occur in a set linear fashion. There are over-lapping stages of development integrated to emerge as existing patterns/pathways. Some of these frequently observed patterns are essential to primal survival and optimizing human performance. Essentially all varieties of patterns are contained in each of the others as an expression element or as a shadow support, a synergistic integration of body-mind as a whole organism. (PC, CP@)

"By working on the movement patterns with the baby as it's developing, you can help the infants on a continuum to have stronger, more balanced alignment, action and integration." (BBC)

A motor engram is a series of processes or commands associated with any cognitive goal or task. With many repetitions entraining a neural pathway, or as patterns emerge with solid hold, an engram may become automated and expressed at the subconscious level. A generalized motor program is a program used to control all movements with a high degree of similarity and the same relative timing. (PC MM)

Each quality of a motor engram is to be activated and enhanced by the growing and adapting child. Each movement pattern is a potential within us. But until we actually do them, they are not accessed and lie dormant or ineffective. This may be an evolutionary carry-over through generations of learned repeated neural laydown, in order to adapt to survive.

Movement is a perception. The first and thus important perception to develop, for survival, is motion/movement based. Each experience a child is exposed to sets the table for efficient quality movement. The developmental sequence is observed in stages to look at characteristics of growth.

Paul Chek (SD, CA) has developed a unique and effective way at evaluating and tracking a child's movement patterns and thus infant development. This is an effective and invaluable tool for guiding youth through life growth. Primal Pattern Development is a very detailed, analytical, and in-depth teaching and clinical tool.

The movements are:

- Twist (breathing; feeling)
- Push (naval radiation; 'no')
- Pull (homologue; 'yes')
- Bend (homo-lateral; adapt)
- Squat-lunge (contra-lateral; hierarchy)
- Gait (walking; destination)

The Primal Pattern Movements are a natural outgrowth of the infant development process. When observing an infant, adolescent, or adult, motor-skills (neural programming), is one way to look at breathing, alignment, balance, tensions, rhythm, and use of space. (PC-CP2)

The real issue is *not* whether you actually witnessed any given stage, but whether the infant's stabilizers and prime moves are working together synergistically. Regardless of how it appears that the infant learns to walk, the only measure of completeness of the infant's growth and development is the integrity of the relevant body systems, which is completely holistic-all inclusive. (PC p. 31 Level 1)

Innate instincts (breathe, reach for breast/mouthing, throwing), serve as evolutionary engrams that aid survival. Nerves myelinate in order of importance for survival. Of the spinal nerves, the motor nerves myelinate before the sensory. In utero vestibular/inner ear (movement in fluid space) is the first to develop, followed by touch to the head (mouth feeding, then taste, smell, hearing and vision. (LH-WBM) This indicates the essential importance of movement-sense for quality growth and development. Infants first learn through the perception of movement, as their senses expand and develop greater acuity.

This process of myelination initiated at the vestibular system, sets up the role the inner ear plays in relationship to later erect posture. The inner ear assists in developing postural tone (the readiness of muscles to respond), an essential element to maintain an upright, efficient and effective posture for work, sport, home. The infant child adapts to one environment of fluid-based (womb), to present to another environment (birth) and initially manage in a horizontal dominant position (lie on back/side/front) to grow into its primary efficient erect posture of verticality. During these growth stages, the three (cervical, thoracic, lumbar) spinal curves develop as neural processes and structural integration.

The infant adjusts, adapts, refines, re-organizes and modifies every sensation and movement to learn to grow and self-perceive and self-manage. It may be useful to expose children to a broad range of stimuli. Experiment with all positions in gravity with children to attain good posture preparation for reaching verticality. This is a simple component that one often is challenged throughout life with. Upon birth, a child is engaged in the fetal position, progressing to outgrowth into a full adult with verticality in posture, until physical death. This is a process in which the body has less levity and gravity disengages the posture until systems collapse. So maintaining functional verticality is important to health and vitality.

The reach and pull motion of the head is (breast feeding, feeling, vision/optic field) not simply to 'stretch' the tissue, but is a change in awareness from outer to inner environment. It is about activating perception - the way a child sees, feels, and ultimately perceives the world it is living in. If in a prone position, the infant manipulates itself, when in the supine body position, the baby manipulates the environment. So it is important to experience a variety of positions and environments.

At all times infant development exercises are integrative and creative. It is a continuum of overlapping growth. These movements develop into primal patterns in adolescents and young adults. One can observe for quality and ease of stability and strength/endurance in performing these effectively.

Work through functional free motion movements such as, gait (walking, track drills, running); squat (lunge, squat, lift overhead, twist); cross pattern (lift, pull patterns, throwing motion). These movements may be done in open play naturally, or as single/group exercise and games. The repetitions, sets, volume and intensity can vary until age ten, but should not be too strenuous, with emphasis on fun and creativity. Once hormonal changes and greater maturity in the teens is initiated there is great need for organized exercise as programming. As the bodily and emotional changes occur during the teen years, a structured program may be designed for effective mental discipline and application of energetic expression and release (sport, dance and weightlifting).

All work or sport movements may be broken down into one of seven key generalized motor programs (neural patterns, engram).

Primal Pattern Movements

1. Squatting
2. Lunging
3. Bending
4. Pushing (open, closed- kinetic chain)
5. Pulling
6. Twisting
7. Gait (walking, running, sprinting).

In essence all movements originate from one of six patterns. Observe the quantity and quality of these primal movements performed in various modes throughout childhood.

Bio-motor ability looks at variables that control capacity or quality of movement to execute a task. Variables included are strength, power, endurance, coordination, speed, balance, agility, flexibility, posture, movements, environments (water, ground, flooring type, air quality) to engage quality postural tone process, pump the circulation, lymphatic and visceral organs and established neural networking for balance brain function. (PC-CP2) These variables are utilized and managed to train a healthy body-mind.

"The more skillful we are, the simpler we become." (PC)

On many levels, the more adept one is at garnering diverse skill-sets (neural engram programming) the better he may advance through life. The potential is unlimited with most children and adults, only tapping the baseline of personal potential for an infinite capacity to learn and grow. The more one experiences, the greater the scope of vision toward realizing even greater experiences and perception potential. Increased and enhanced perception yields enhanced power.

Parental Suggestion

Allow the infant periods of time twice a day, as far away from feeding as possible, to lie on his stomach so hey can learn to explore the usage through stretching of different muscle groups. This also assists in strengthening the neck muscles as he learns to lift his head. The parent can also gently move the infant's limbs (making sure that the baby seems to enjoy this) back and forth and in small circles manually. Four or five repetitions of each movement are advised. Pay careful attention that this does not seem to cause any distress.

Learning to Grow

You must grow to learn and learn to grow. It takes growth to change and change to grow.

Throughout life, learning, growth and change are active variables. Many individuals take some time, reflection, self-realization and awareness to know how they best learn. Some learn, adapt and modify their behavior to manage at a different pace. There are different styles of learning that are frequently ingrained at an early age.

"50% of ability to learn is developed in the first four years of life and another 30% by age 8." (The Learning Revolution; *Gordon Dryden and Jeanette Vos).*

At birth the child is untapped consciousness. It has an unlimited potential for higher intelligence due to expanded consciousness. It is throughout life that the growing child becomes contracted and often conflicted in body-mind, until an awakening, enlightening expansion is experienced. To maintain balanced body-mind is of prime importance in achieving higher health and attained higher consciousness with integrated body, mind and spirit.

"If you have a big enough dream or idea, then you do not need negativity. Allow your child to have a new dream connection daily." (RCM)

Recognizing and addressing varied learning styles in children provides validation, confidence and security in their individual process, allowing them to experience, learn and grow. It is important to learn how you learn. Throughout life, many do not look at their self and how they may individually interact in the world. Learn how you best respond in certain situations, what you like/dislike and what is serving you. Learn how your brain is trained or how it operates (i.e. a memory recall, imagery, language, cognition emotional response), and how to effectively become a free thinker.

The human brain form has undergone evolutionary changes over time to survive, adapt and morph into the appropriate functional capacity. There are divisions of the brain that develop at different times. The reptilian brain (lower) begins its function in the first trimester of gestation. The old mammalian brain (middle) in the second trimester, while the neo-cortex/neo-mammalian brain (upper ~ 'human brain') in the third trimester, followed by pre-frontal cortex (pre-frontal lobes; cognition) develops after birth. Biologist Bruce Lipton (*Biology of Belief*) observed how the first cell created by nature was in effect a brain unto itself and a template that underlies all subsequent development. Maybe it is a holographic representation of 'self' to be enhanced, projected and propagated into higher life-forms and intelligence of being.

Reptile Brain (lower self) ~ ID (survival, react and protect
Mammalian Brain   ~ Ego (emotional, cognitive)
Neo-mammalian Brain   ~ Conscious awareness dreaming,
  (higher self)   intuition

Memes are self replicating packages of information that propagate themselves across the ecologies of mind in a pattern of reproduction similar to a virus. Memes reproduce themselves and interact with their surroundings. (SD) Memes infect and influence the mind, via thoughts, ideas and lifestyle practices.

Memes are set in social conditioning and programming that may affect an individual or group on many levels. Memetics is the study of language. The young growing child is open to learning much in the process of growth and development into maturity. The young child is also open and susceptible to many varieties of great influences. Models and modes of learning of the greatest influence is the parents, school, social groups (i.e. religion, teams, clubs). Children often learn by modeling or imitating another person or thing. It is important to consider who is modeling who?

Memetic discussion is an effort to expose the connection between the ideas (themes, trends, views), carried in, the underlying thinking systems, value systems, world views and coping systems. (SD) This concept may seem benign in effect, but the subtle nature of an active meme or engram (be it volitional conscious or unconscious), may have deep socio-cultural impact on the physical-emotional well-being of an individual or group.

"90% of people do not evolve their mind past age 12. Everything they know is often learned by age 12." (PC)

Some children learn on their own; others in groups, diverse settings, in interactive/private, or divisional/integrative modes. This diversity also modifies as one learns and experiences more. During infant development, it is said that the brain makes 50% of the main brain cell connections, the pathways for all future learning. (TLR). Great influence for learning is initiated at home. Early home education provides the largest body of learning and carries great impact. This is an influential period of movement (motor-learning) and brain (intellectual/academic learning). Thus parent education and awareness training may be important to consider pre- birth and post- birth.

In many cases the education system, or other forms of provided education and environment hold back children from learning at a more rapid rate, and hinder their personal potential and ability to learn, grow and develop. It is important to provide freedom to learn with different learning styles in diverse settings.

There are different types of intelligence that develop throughout life. There is social intelligence (ability to socio-culturally interact), emotional intelligence (ability to react/respond with emotional integrity and stability), physical intelligence (ability to move gracefully), cognitive intelligence (ability to think, problem-solve.

There are 7 intelligence centers described by Gardner (Howard Gardner; Harvard Professor Psychologist, *The Learning Revolution*):
- linguistic
- mathematical-logic
- visual/spatial
- musical
- inter-personal (social skills; relate with others)
- intra-personal (reflective; know self)
- bodily-physical.

The brain also has hemispheric dominance over select stimuli and response activity. The left and right side of the two hemispheres of the brain are separated by the corpus collosum. All responses, either reflexive or learned are neurally wrapped through specific developments or experiences.

BRAIN HEMISPHERE:

Left	Right
- logic	- rhyme
- words	- rhythm
- numbers	- music
- mathematics	- pictures
- sequence	- imagination

Elementary school education programs focus often on two faculties; linguistic (ability to speak, read, write) and logical (logic, reasoning, math, science). (TLR) This practice limits the learning experience to only two (linguistic, math/logic) of the 7 intelligence centers, and appears to be dominant in left brain activity. This predominant bias toward left-brain activity may restrict or inhibit right-brain activity for freedom for creativity to aid complete early childhood development. Since creative freedom is an important characteristic in early development, the balance of right and left brain activity is crucial. Right-brain (creativity, art) is often limited/restricted in home and school time. Some believe that the impact of previous years exposure to logical programming and early training may be best served in natural school practices and not introduce computer, math until later childhood years. This may engage varied social development traits and greater brain hemispheric balance, resulting in an individual being more mature and complete in later years.

The three most common learning styles are:
- heptic learners ('moving along', kinesthetic, tactile; feel body move)
- visual (see pictures, use imagery) (TLR, p.131)
- auditory (listening, sound).

"95% of all education taught at schools around the world, is taught in the mathematical-logic learning style. Only 5-8% of population learn in this manner. (PC)

People exhibit a combination of learning styles, with one or two dominant learning styles proving to be most effective. Most commonly practiced is visual learning (see; imagery, artist), then audible (hear; musician), kinesthetic (feel; athlete dancer), and least common mathematical-logic (cognitive; scientist).

It is observed that most students learn best by moving and adults have a more visual preference. Yet most school programs (teaching and testing) are based on mathematical logic learning style. This may fail to recognize all the parts that make up whole intelligence, and leave a learning deficiency.

Because infants are more motor-sensory; (learn by motion), and adults are sensory-motor (prefer visual). Kinesthesis, the ability to learn by feeling as one moves (neural-tactile sense) is the most commonly utilized learning modality when young, while visual is common with adults and most having two predominant learning styles.

Some keys to effective learning are: be in the moment; be present (body-mind centered; learn your way; open mind ~ open hearing (increase capacity potential); relaxed alertness (still body and quiet mind); awake and alert (focused and calm); create connection (your story or view); open communication; rest and regeneration.

Ask: How do you like/best to learn? How do you want to be shown or taught?

Show me…

Explain it…

Let me try it…

"Even fifteen minutes of rocking, rubbing, rolling and stroking a premature baby four times a day will greatly help its ability to coordinate movements and therefore to learn." (LH)

Parental Suggestion

Most children develop an early proclivity to access the world through either hearing, seeing, or feeling as primary input source. This is primarily due to early life's experiences and parental influence. The emphasis on one sensory pathway of input over another gives a slanted view of the world and omits at least

two-thirds of environmental input for the child. It is crucial for parents, during the first four years of development, to allow the child to experience multiple different pleasing sounds: In nature – children should be exposed to:
- various complexities of music from the lullaby to the operatic),
- smells (a few drops of therapeutic essential oils on the bottom of their feet at night will expose them to fragrance, but the subtler smells of fruits and plants are also needed),
- feeling (not only tactile experiences but encouraging them to share how things make them feel), and
- visual (help them see the subtleties of color by counting how many colors of green they see in the park, and learning to differentiate form by spotting birds and animals in their natural habitat).

It is the child who has omni-sensory perception who experiences the full enjoyment of life.

Children learn best by doing. This allows them to use a combination of their faculties to learn or accomplish a task Allow them the freedom to play, create and express themselves. There are different types of intelligence that develop through life. There is social (ability to socio-culturally interact), emotional intelligence (ability to respond and react with emotional integrity and stability), physical intelligence, (ability to move gracefully), cognitive intelligence (ability to think, problem-solve).

Parental Suggestion

To learn how to integrate information beyond the shallow understandings of the face value of appearances, right brain (non-cognitive accessing of information) and left brain (cognitive accessing) need to be smoothly integrated in their functions. Parents can promote this in toddlers by playing games that cross the limbs over one another. Additionally, ambidexterity should be encouraged in children.

Learn to play - play to learn

"Playfulness is a measure of intelligence." (Osho)

If children do not have the freedom to play, they often do not have the freedom to develop intelligence. It takes courage (create change and get out of box), heart (effort and compassion), creative instinct ~ intuition, (ability to allow for expansion of higher health). Many think of intelligence as being restricted to a mental quality/faculty, but intelligence is truly multi-faceted. Existing high intelligence is of diverse make-up.

Instinct is the foundation for genius. This is creative freedom and ultimately intention to access greater potential. Creativity nourishes self-esteem (play, explore, re-create). Instincts emerge from our sub-conscious mind, which is said to account for 92% of our individual consciousness totality. (PC-CP).

One may be approximately only 8% consciously awake and aware, leaving a larger portion to automated acts, a seemingly passive process that elicits outcome responses that may or may not save the individual. Raise conscious children. Provide safe and secure environment. Allow them freedom to be.

"Children need to be less like adults and paradoxically, adults need to be more like children. More fun and less stress!" (RCM)

Parental Suggestion

Parents often think that they need to make their children aware of all possible dangers and hostilities that could befall them. This gives them the socially conditioned view of the adult instead of the natural light-hearted spontaneity of the child. It is a form of faithlessness not to allow the child's inner guidance to express.

By all means, safeguard your child, but in a way that will not even communicate to them what you are doing. To give them worldviews of danger is to attract it. To quote the philosopher

James Allen: *"As a man thinketh in his heart, so is he."* Shakespeare said in *Julius Caesar, "That which I feared is come upon me."*

Don't protect your child from a scraped knee but don't allow them to be in danger of falling off the balcony, is a sound philosophy. The bumps and scrapes of life, mental and emotional, create robustness. Strive to allow your child to see his own answers through your gentle guidance rather than having parenthood become a dictatorship.

Play and recreation time may be turned into a learning experience, and learning can be viewed as play. Make a connection to the event, be it home, school, sport, work. Use of linking tools may aid moving, imagination and creativity. These reach deeper levels of the mind for greater retention upon learning.

"People of all ages can learn virtually anything if allowed to do it through their own unique styles, their own personal strength." (Gordon Dryden, Jeanette Vos, The Learning Revolution, *p.98) (Barbara Proshing in* Diversity is our Strength.*)*

A relaxed state is best for activating long term memory. There is also close anatomical reference with the emotional centre close to long term memory. (TLR). This may be why a child or adult experiences an emotional event that registers with higher significance in memory. This could be an important observation. Many are consciously and unconsciously aware of recessed deep traumas or significant events that may not be recognized, addressed, or comprehended.

With trauma (physical/emotional) there is often an energetic disruption in the physical and subtle energetic bodies (physical/etheric/emotional/causal bodies represented). There could be an energy 'block' (accumulated life-force) or energy 'leak' (too much life-force out). Often with a traumatic or stimulating event, there is an 'energy pattern hold' at the physical (structural) level or emotional, mental level). Less divided life force energy allows for enhanced health and performance.

This may need to be addressed by a medical or holistic health professional. This is very relevant as trauma, wounds, injury or illness experienced by a developing youth may be carried through life, while creating inhibition, pain and dysfunction.

> *"True knowledge is that which overcomes fear. Increase knowledge of self. Experience is a process in which knowledge is synthesized into wisdom."* (PC)

Fear is set in ancient survival systems, as an instinct to avoid harm (JCP.'02). This is at the root of human behavior, and in many young children and adults may be layered with compiled experiences throughout life. This may show in body language, posture, breathing quality, movement restrictions, mental outlook holding patterns and general vitality. Learn what works for you and when. Find what serves your health and well-being best.

To play is to freely express one's self. Play should have safe guidelines, but avoid rigid rules, that may restrict creative freedom. Play may include: freedom to think and move; fun, curiosity, spontaneity, adventure, re-create, discovery, creativity ...

Children have a great range of energy displayed as enthusiasm and curiosity. They generally want to feel and see, to learn and experience the world as their immediate environment. All internal conflict is produced by fear of possible harm or the unknown, fear of change in not knowing what the process or resulting outcome is. Children often display less apprehension when exposed to a new experience. They are less conditioned (programmed response), so less inhibition and 'fear' programming is demonstrated.

Many young people may seem awake in that they are not physically sleeping, but the quality of mental alertness varies. Some may be non-alert (i.e. lack quality sleep, blood sugar management, hydration, lack emotional connection), and some hyper-active physically and mentally (adrenal drain, hemispheric brain balance, over-stimulated neuro-hormonal system, electromagnetic pollution/interference).

An important element of practice is to be 'in your body' (physical preparation and awareness), and to maintain an open mind, (to have fun and perform at your best).

Some continue to press the limits of the physical body (i.e. extreme sports). They may perform like uninhibited children 'not knowing better' or mentally block out the negative and execute the positive outcome. This is a tricky dilemma with the high level of risk-reward. It may be that the performer is highly skilled, has good mental control and exhibits 'performance ease'. Congruency of body, mind and spirit allows for the greatest health and performance potential. On the other hand what some children and performers alike may learn consciously/sub-consciously to do or entrain themselves is to be is 'out of their body' (not physically aware) and 'closed mind' (out of touch mentally). In this scenario, there may be less than optimal opportunity for safe and quality execution of a task, or less chance of longevity and repeatability of performance.

Performance ease is akin being in 'the zone'. The zone is a term referred to when performance is executed flawlessly, with little physical-mental effort and just 'felt good' - 'being in the moment.' This is a parameter that many performers try to achieve and repeat.

A child should be taught how to be in the moment to enjoy life, and be in the moment to move as he progresses toward achieving optimal potential throughout life. Children may have to adapt their individual needs to survive and excel, but parents should avoid or manage the stress presented during their early years. To be healthy and happy, a child must be aware of what makes them happy and feel good. Children should enjoy life and have fun in expressing themselves in the process of learning, growth and development.

Parental Suggestion

Children who are subjected to parents living vicariously through them because they have abandoned themselves, live in the stress of parental expectations. When parents value accomplishments and achievements rather than inner victories and overcomings, this becomes an emphasis in their rearing. Many little ones from the age of three onward go from one class to another, their days filled with having to learn, do and know, instead of enjoyment. Children subjected to the constant need to prove their cognitive and other abilities may become achievers, but develop A-type, highly stressed personalities. In the footsteps of their parents they abandon themselves, hardly knowing what makes their hearts sing. Abandonment of self is the origin of all addiction and the source of unhappiness and ill health. Support your child's passion and allow him or her much leisure time to learn the highly-prized skills few adults possess – to know ourselves and be comfortable in our own company.

Growth and Development Stages

The critical developmental stages that once missed and cannot be reclaimed can be encouraged into full development by the appropriate activity types as given below. For example, all children develop a skill of producing a map from a journey or a proposed journey at the age of twelve. Developing the proper mind-body coordination appropriate for that age will assist in refining the ability to produce such a map. Even though all children of all races develop the ability at the same time, the skill level will vary and can be enhanced by physical activity.

Age	Experience	Activity Type
1. Conception –10 mos.	In utero, fluid dynamics, shared-assisted feeding and consciousness	Clean, quality nutrition & thoughts (early parenting)
2. Birth 0–1 years	Infant level	Feel to move and breathe
3. 0–3 years	'I-ness' (self-aware as individual ego separate from mother; explore self and environment)	Creative and open play
4. 3–7 years	Early movement (integrated exposure to diverse movement types)	Broad range movement and thinking; specialized skill-set (dance, sport)
5. 7–12 years	Neuro-plastic (programmed movement/emotions of body-mind)	Stability for mobility (posture, form and function)
6. 12–18 years	Teenage (neuro-hormonal, gender difference)	Independent (emotional-hormonal growth expression
7. 18–21 years	Neural growth maturity; relationship with self and others	Balanced WO/WI (work ~ rest ratio)

(Free open play → creative games → skill acquisition → organized sport (team and individual) competitions (goals, to high performance program design).

Balance Work-In (WI) and Work-Out (WO) Practices

Work In Energy in	Work Out Energy out
That which is performed without excess stress - (heart Rate breathe, digestion monitored)	Stress load capacity, volume intensity margins monitored
Rest, relax, regenerate, rejuvenate, cultivate and accumulate life-force energy	Stimulate growth/training effect
Mental Fitness	Physical Fitness
Anabolic – builds body	Catabolic – breaks down body
Initiate at all ages	Free motion, body weight train medicine. ball, swiss balls
Breathing, postural control, Balance/walking	No external wts. until structural/hormonal development
Yoga/meditation	Develop in teens w/professional program design
Tai-chi (light martial arts) Dance forms	Individual and team sport activity and sport-specific training and conditioning

Variables
Work In:
- Breath pattern steady
- Stillness (mental focus and emptiness)
- Visual activity (internal/external vision)
- Varied subtle stimulus (music, toning, micro frequency modulation)
- Nature (organic interaction)

Work Out:
- Aerobic/anaerobic switch; core control; endurance
- Strength, power, endurance combo
- Rest - work ratio

- full body movements, rhythm, breathe quality, control stability and posture (form)
- cross-pattern.

Work toward desired goals and optimal health and performance. Achieve physical and mental fitness to meet the required needs.

The more complex a movement or skill-set execution, the greater the importance the fundamental early development of a child. There is a cumulative affect of varied individual experiences and exposures that develop the psycho-sontic makeup of a growing child.

Chart A

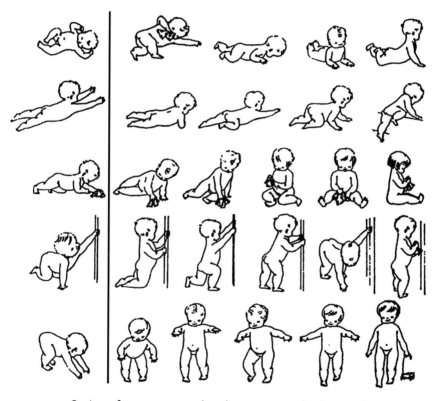

Series of gross motor development on the basis of
self-induced movements (from Pikler 1972).

These are estimated guidelines as stages. There is no one path that all individuals follow, but individual characteristics with a shared foundation. These stages are not distinct and overlap and integrate in g and d.

* If concerns seek medication from professional or holistic health consultant.

Chart B

Primal Pattern® Development

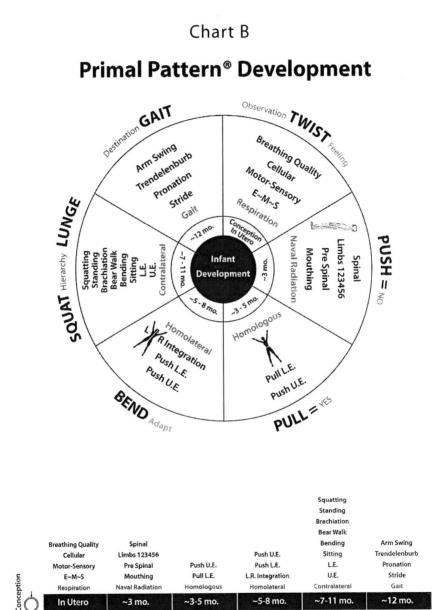

Conception	In Utero	~3 mo.	~3-5 mo.	~5-8 mo.	~7-11 mo.	~12 mo.
	Breathing Quality	Spinal			Squatting	
	Cellular	Limbs 123456			Standing	
	Motor-Sensory	Pre Spinal			Brachiation	
	E~M~S	Mouthing	Push U.E.	Push U.E.	Bear Walk	Arm Swing
	Respiration	Naval Radiation	Pull L.E.	Push L.E.	Bending	Trendelenburb
			Homologous	L.R. Integration	Sitting	Pronation
				Homolateral	L.E.	Stride
					U.E.	Gait
					Contralateral	

Progressively work into greater complexity in movement and thinking (creativity, problem solving, cognition).

Observe the 'movement ease' of a child. Look at the fluid flow of smooth sequential motor programming and the emotional energy attached to the event. Observe breathe, posture, balance, stability, strength, endurance, power, skill as a child progresses through bi-motor accumulation (neural network).

Contra-lateral movement (opposite limb coordination) underlies the integration of all three (sagital, fintal, transverse) planes of movement and spirallic movement. Observe for this transition in effective movement possible and faulty movement patterns, biomechic faults, structural restrictions and breakdown in quality of 'form' and exertion of a task.

• Importance of full body-mind integration to illicit a quality response and desired performance. 'Anything the mind can conceive the body can achieve.' Have a full relationship of body-mind.
• Global full body movement
• Cross – midline of body (Right and Left brain)
• Use Left and Right hand equally.

References

Chek, Paul; *C.H.E.K Practitioner Level – 1*; C.H.E.K Institute; Vista, CA.

Chek, Paul; *C.H.E.K Holistic Lifestyle Coach, Level 3*; C.H.E.K Institute; Vista, CA.

Chek, Paul; *How to Eat, Move and Be Healthy*; C.H.E.K Institute, Publication, 2004.

Chek, Paul; *Movement That Matters*; C.H.E.K. Institute, Vista, CA. 2001.

Cohen, Bonnie Bainbridge; *The Evolutionary Origins of Movement*; Amhurst, MA, 1986.

Hartley, Linda; *Wisdom of the Body Moving*; North Atlantic Books, Berkley, CA, 1995.

Pert, Candice; *Molecules of Emotion*; Simon and Shuster; New York, NY, 1999.

Dryden, Gordon and Vos, Jeanette; *The Learning Web Ltd*; Auckland, NZ, 1997.

Sandow, Eugene; *Life is Movement*; The National Health Press; London, UK, 1929.

Beck, Don Edward; Cowan, Christopher C.; *Spiral Dynamics*; Blackwell Publishing; Malden, Ma, 2005.

Pearce, Joseph Chilton; *The Biology of Transcendence*; Park Street Press; Vermont, 2002.

Lipton, Bruce; *Biology of Belief*; Mountain of Love/Elite Books; Santa Rosa, CA, 2005.

Blythe, Sally Goddard; *The Well Balanced Child*; Hawthorn Press, Gloucestershire, UK, 2004.

CLOSING

Our world is our school and our fellow creatures our teachers. All around us the environment speaks to us, wanting to share its mysteries in ecstatic revelations.

The greatest gifts we can give our children are the intangibles of life: the robust self-confidence to ride its crests and valleys, the humble awareness of its magic.

It is well to encourage our babies to reach with exploring fingers for their teddy today and the world tomorrow. But the prevailing impressions come from our examples. We cannot instill happiness in our children if we are a stranger to it ourselves.

The desire to give to them by example the knowledge that life is good and beautiful can be the catalyst for our shedding of the cobwebs of care-worn attitudes. In this way our children also become our teachers, showing us once again the forgotten art of a life of grand adventure and graceful fluidity born of trust.

Bonus Section

Homeopathic-spagyric Medications for a More Comprehensive Home Apothecary

"The human body has one ability not possessed by any machine – the ability to repair itself."

—George E. Crile, Jr., Medical Doctor

"To prepare for the worst is to have the luxury of expecting the best."

—Almine

HOMEOPATHIC-SPAGYRIC MEDICATIONS FOR A MORE COMPREHENSIVE HOME APOTHECARY

Over the years of home-treating my children and the many visitors to our home when they were unwell, I have relied heavily on a more comprehensive method of dealing with disease; homeopathic-spagyric medications. Tried and tested, I would be remiss if I did not share this treasure trove with you.[19]

Pekana Homeopathic-spagyric Medications

Pekana homeopathic-spagyric medications dramatically accelerate the body's immune response and healing processes. They also stimulate production of vital enzymes that play a decisive role in metabolism and immuno-biological reactions and act as natural antimicrobials. In addition, these high-energy remedies help damaged organ tissues function efficiently again, which improves the excretion of endogenic and exogenic toxins – the basis of many chronic illnesses – lodged in the organs and connective tissues. Furthermore, this type of holistic therapy causes no microbial resistance and produces no negative side effects.

What are spagyrics?

First developed by the 16th century Swiss physician and alchemist Paracelsus, spagyrism represents a form of homeopathy in which both vital healing energy and active substances are extracted from medicinal plants, creating powerful mother tinctures that can be further potentized. Derive from the Greek words *spao* (separate) and *ageiro* (unite), the term spagyric means to take something apart and then re-unite it.

Paracelsus pointed out that the vital energy of an herb is more important than the plant material itself. Spagyric remedies were originally created by putrefying parts of wild herbs, then distilling

---

19 All are available by calling 502 499 0016 or, toll-free, 877 552 5646.

the material in a special device to produce concentrated, high alcohol (70-80%) aromatic solutions. The extracted bulk plant matter was dried and burned to an ash. Finally, this unpurified ash was recombined with the solution. As a result, the finished spagyric essence contained the mineral constituent parts of the plant.

This original method had some serious drawbacks. Modern yeasts were unavailable 500 years ago and therefore the alchemists could not use today's fermentation techniques. Instead they were forced to distill the plant materials, which destroyed important ingredients such as alkaloids, vitamins and enzymes. Moreover the old method simply combined untreated ash with the solution, which mean the final remedies often contained impurities.

What makes Pekana homeopathic-spagyric medications unique for detoxification, regeneration and restoration?

Modified through the ages, the spagyric process has been greatly refined by Pekana founder and owner Dr. Peter Beyersdorff, who holds a doctorate in pharmacy. The modern manufacturing method developed by Pekana is unique in the world today and results in homeopathic-spagyric medications of exceptional quality and efficacy. All remedies are produced at the company's Kisslegg, Germany facility according to Good Manufacturing Practices (GMP) certification.

Pekana homeopathic-spagyric medications capture the entire living essence of healing plants. Listed in the Homeopathic Pharmacopeia (HAB), the spagyric processing method developed by master pharmacist Dr. Beyersdorff produces medications with both powerful energetic and biochemical effects. The combinations of spagyrically processed herbs, synergistic minerals and homeopathic substances are peerless in their capacity to help the body eliminate toxins and restore proper physiological function.

The process starts by fermenting selected herbs into what is essentially a wine using special yeasts and sugars. Each herb produces its own unique alcohol and other fermentation products. Therefore the resulting product is alive and composed of a complex blend of metabolic products compatible with the energy (qi) of the plant.

In Chinese medicine terms, this step could be looked upon as developing the 'yin' of the plant. It is completely different from adding alcohol to an herb to extract its components.

Next the tincture is purified through a series of filtration steps, while the leftover plant residue is burned to an ash. This develops the most 'yang' quality of the plant. The ash is placed in a filter tube within a water solution until clear, pure crystals form, indicating the maximum amount of the minerals have been extracted.

In the last step, Pekana reunites the mineral filtrate with the tincture. This combination of the fully developed yin with the fully developed yang results in a complete product, the spagyric medicine. All the color and aroma of the remedy forms during this reunification process.

The spagyric medicine is then made into a homeopathic medicine by hand succession. Hand succession is extremely important in that it adds another element of focused human intent into the production process.

Finally up to eight homeopathic-spagyric single ingredients are blended together to form the complete Pekana remedy. A single ingredient would provide a valuable medicine but combining eight components creates a remedy that will have a broad spectrum of action in a wide variety of case presentations.

Pekana employees carry out this incredibly sophisticated spagyric process in a family-like work environment. All products are made according to Good Manufacturing Practices standards and certification, which ensures that the ingredients have not been contaminated by microbes or metal toxins. This certification is difficult to obtain. The combination of good science and traditional craftsmanship comes through in the finished product.

What is particularly exceptional about Pekana remedies is that they are often well tolerated even by patients hypersensitive to alcohol in tinctures. This possibly results from the unique fermentation process. Pekana medications contain alcohol, but it is primarily part of the broad spectrum of metabolic products from fermentation rather than something added as a solvent.

Pekana facts

- Produced by a unique spagyric processing method listed in the German Homeopathic Pharmacopeia (HAB).
- GMP-certified to ensure the highest production standards for quality, safety and efficacy.
- Combination formulas made from fresh plants or dried herbs prescribed in the Homeopathic Pharmacopeia that Pekana analyzes and standardizes to maintain constantly high product quality.
- Filtered, never distilled, to keep the effective substances intact and ensure that alkaloids, enzymes and vitamins are not destroyed.
- Formulas cleans the extracellular matrix to promote effective excretion of toxins and transport of essential molecules.
- Hand-succussed to maintain vital energy.
- FDA-listed and supported by clinical application studies.
- High energy content verified by comparative chromatography.
- Received award for innovation from the State of Baden-Wurttemberg for Exemplary Achievement and Performance.

TREATING YOUR CHILD WITH HOMEOPATHIC-SPAGYRIC REMEDIES

(See dosages at the end of this section. Unless otherwise noted, products are liquid, administered in drops.)

1. Allergies

Pro-aller	for allergies
Toxex	general excretion
apo-Hepat	· liver function

For food allergies add:

apo-Stom	stomach and intestinal function
Opsonat	mucus membrane inflammation

For skin allergies add:

Itires	lymphatic drainage (good for acne)
Dercut	skin diseases

2. Asthma and chest congestion

Bronchi-pertu syrup	asthma and whooping cough
apo-Infekt	bacterial and viral infections
Opsonat	focal infections, mucus membranes

(Asthma suffers should blow up several balloons each day to strengthen muscles used in exhaling.)

3. Bronchial Infections – including bronchitis/pneumonia

apo-Pulm expectorant syrup - bronchial congestion
OR

apo-tuss	coughs, laryngitis, hoarseness

AND
apo-Infekt
Opsonat

4. Cancer

The full detoxification program given on www.belvaspata.com must be used to restore a derailed system such as that of a cancer patient. Also use Viscum drops for tumors.

5. Diabetes

Speci-chol	pancreatic disturbances
apo-Hepat	liver function
Toxex	excretion of heavy metals
Opsonat	focal infections, mucous membrane infections

6. Headaches, migraines, joint, limb, nerve pain

apo-Dolor	headaches, migraines
Opsonat	focal infections
Itires	lymph function

Have a pediatric chiropractor check for a subluxation in the neck, especially the axis and atlas. A blow from a ball can cause the skull to be crooked on the atlas which in turn could be the cause of teeth grinding (this could also be from parasites).

7. Herpes and chicken pox

Dercut	skin disease
apo-Infekt	bacterial and viral infections

8. Hypertension and mood swings

Psy-Stabil	psychological disturbances/fears
Coro-calm	cardiac sedative; anxiety

9. Insomnia

Somcupin	sleep disturbances
Coro-calm	anxiety

10. Measles, rubella, scarlet fever

Dercut lotion/drops	skin diseases
apo-Infekt	viral or bacterial infections

11. Mumps
    Itires drops/ointment lymphatic drainage

12. Rhinitis and sinusitis
    Ricura   rhinitis, sinusitis
    Itires   lymphatic drainage
    apo-Infekt   viral or bacterial infections

13. Tonsillitis, laryngitis
    Septonsil   tonsillitis, sore throat
    apo-Infekt   viral and bacterial infection
    Opsonat   mucous membrane inflammation

14. Urinary tract infections
    Akutur   urological infections
    Akutur medicinal tea urological infections
    Renelix   kidney function

How to use the Pekana Remedies

• Administer them as far from meals as possible.
• Don't bring them into contact with metals – use a plastic teaspoon.
• The use of mint, menthol, camphor and eucalyptus in conjunction with these remedies will inhibit their proper functioning.
• They can be used **all together** in the bottom of a glass with a bit of pure water.
• Drinking lots of water as these remedies eliminate toxins and is essential to avoid a healing crisis.
• For long term conditions, use for 90 days.

Recommended Dosages for Children

(Away from meals)

apo-Dolor
School Children: 10–15 drops 3–4 times per day
Small Children: 5–8 drops 3–4 times per day

Akutur
School Children: 10-15 drops 3 times per day directly or in liquid
Small Children: 5 drops 3 times per day

apo-Hepat
School Children: 7–10 drops 3 times per day
Small Children: 5 drops 3 times per day

apo-Infekt
School Children: 7–10 drops 3 times per day
Small Children: 5 drops 3 times per day

apo-Pulm
School Children: 1 tsp 5-7 times per day

apo-Stom
School Children: 7–10 drops 3 times per day
Small Children: 5 drops 3 times per day

Bronchi-Pertu
School Children: 1 tsp 5-7 times per day

coro-Calm
School Children: 7–10 drops 3 times per day
Small Children: 5 drops 3 times per day

Dercut
School Children: 7–10 drops 3 times per day
Small Children: 5 drops 3 times per day

Itires
School Children: 7–10 drops 3 times per day
Small Children: 5 drops 3 times per day

Opsonat
School Children: 7–10 drops 3 times per day
Small Children: 5 drops 3 times per day

Proaller
School Children: 7–10 drops 3 times per day
Small Children: 5 drops 3 times per day

Psy-Stabil
School Children: 10-15 drops 3-4 times per day

Radinex
School Children: 10 drops 2-3 times per day

Renelix
School Children: 7–10 drops 3 times per day
Small Children: 5 drops 3 times per day

Ricura
School Children: 7–10 drops 3 times per day
Small Children: 5 drops 3 times per day

Septonsil
School Children: 7–10 drops 3 times per day
Small Children: 5 drops 3 times per day

Somcupin
School Children: 7–10 drops 3 times per day
Small Children: 5 drops 3 times per day

Speci-Chol
School Children: 7–10 drops 3 times per day
Small Children: 5 drops 3 times per day

Toxex
School Children: 7–10 drops 3 times per day
Small Children: 5 drops 3 times per day

Viscum
School Children: 7–10 drops 3 times per day
Small Children: 5 drops 3 times per day

Appendices

I. THE LANGUAGE OF PAIN

At a spiritual level, all illness, pain, disease, and injuries are the language of Spirit telling us what aspect of our lives needs to be brought into harmony with who we are. Therefore, it is wise to examine what is behind the symptom and ask for the lesson, then embrace it and release it. When we release core issues, the illness, pain or disease goes away.

If there is no need for the language of pain to get our attention, we won't become sick. Nobody causes another person to get sick. A sickness that is labeled contagious certainly has the potential to spread, but it cannot invade the body if we are balanced and have healthy boundaries. The only time a germ or virus slips in, is if we have forsaken ourselves by suppressing the subpersonalities or engaging in self- deprecating thoughts or beliefs. We become immune to disease when we balance the emotional body and we are home for ourselves by reconnecting the subpersonalities and allowing them freedom of expression.

Accidents don't occur to those who walk in balance. If we have no cause for an accident to manifest, we will walk in grace, even if we are in the center of an earthquake or hurricane. The language of pain includes injuries from accidents, because in truth, there is no such thing as an accident. We masterfully manifested the incident.

If pain is the language of Spirit, what is the language of the soul? It is our feelings. When we have done something that feels wonderful, we have just lived our highest truth. If we follow our feelings, we automatically walk our highest truth.

Note: Spirit as used in this context, pertains to our Highest Self as a being as vast as the cosmos. It is when we aren't remembering this true identity that disease occurs. Soul, on the other hand, relates to our Higher Self, our fourth-dimensional aspect that has designed our assignments for this life. It communicates the assignments to our higher bodies, which in turn communicates it to our emotional body (assuming the mental body lets these messages through). Then it is felt in the heart.

We must be careful when it comes to feelings, though, because fears can masquerade as feelings. Feelings are also frequently confused with emotions. I would like to clarify this so when we are analyzing the language of pain, we know the difference.

Feelings vs. Emotions

Feeling is a way to access information that isn't accessible to reason. It bypasses the mind. Therefore, feeling is a non cognitive way of getting information, which registers as an intuitive knowing. Feeling is the right brain accessing the unknown. It deals with things beyond the five senses and logic. Emotion has as its foundation, desire.

How to Deal with Pain: When experiencing a painful situation, don't analyze it while you are feeling the initial emotion. That clouds judgment. Just experience the emotion. Afterwards, when you are calm and can access the feeling without it being colored by emotion, then use your left brain and see intuition behind the appearances so you can embrace the lesson. (If we are tangled up in emotions, we may miss the core lesson and then we have to create a similar circumstance later.)

To change our emotions, we need to alter our perception. It works in reverse too, because altering emotion causes altered perception. The two work hand-in-hand.

It is necessary for the sake of clarity to explain the different meanings of the word love: Divine love is a state of being that remains when all fear is removed. Love can also be the desire to include, which makes it an emotion. Love can also be a vibration in the cells that resonates with the intent of the universe. And the intent of the universe is to include all of creation within itself. Divine love is unconditional.

We don't need to worry about how to generate it because we already are love. Simply remove all fear by seeing behind the appearances and the filter obstructing love will be removed.

Sentimental love is a joyous emotion that results from believing that another completes us. We may choose a partner who brings in what we don't have, or haven't developed yet, or have given away. Consequently, in his or her presence we experience wholeness. It is a false sense of wholeness, but it can elicit joy. That explains why some people feel they have no identity away from the union as a couple. The same feeling of joy that results from sentimental love, can be developed within ourselves by balancing our emotional aspects.

Compassion is a response of empathy to another's emotions and the subsequent interpretation of it. Unlike divine love, the compassionate response to another changes as perception alters, taking on different forms along the rungs of enlightenment.

Interpreting the Language of Pain

The following list of body parts and symptoms will assist us in recognizing the areas of our lives that are out of balance when symptoms manifest.

General areas and systems of the body

Breath indicates our ability to express ourselves in life. If we don't express ourselves, it is as though someone has placed a boulder on our chest and we cannot fully breathe. Frequently, people place the boulder on themselves.

The breath is expressing our life force, so **asthma** patients have life force problems. Often they were stifled from expressing as children. Babies and toddlers know the big picture of who they are, so they may experience tremendous frustration over being trapped in a physical body, unable to express the glory of their true identity. It is helpful to assist children to find safe avenues to explore their gifts and talents. When the life force becomes suppressed, the exhaling process becomes difficult, as is the case with asthma.

The **fluids** of our body have to do with emotions. **Blood**, in particular, is the equivalent of love. The ability to love is very important. If we deliberately withhold love we find constriction in our arteries. **Hardened arteries** mean hardened emotions and condition of love.

The **heart** has to do with giving love. Drawing love from the limitless supply of the universe it should flow out through our heart. If we close our heart because of fear or from not being fully present in our body, then we begin to give energy from our life force center. This depletes us.

In order to insulate ourselves from this drain of energy, a layer of fat could build up around the solar plexus (stomach area). Light workers frequently have this layer of fat as an attempt to protect their energy source. People who suffered childhood abuse may use **fat** to insulate themselves from other people.

It is important to live fully in the body. Many people have suffered childhood sexual abuse and learned to leave the body when things got unpleasant. If we don't stay in the body and feel, then the heart center remains closed and we cannot fulfill our highest calling on this planet.

Soft tissues and ligaments reflect attitudes. Is our attitude positive? Do we frequently complain? The **joints** have to do with how flexible we are. The soft tissues control the joints, so they are affected too. For example, in the past, prior to a seminar I would receive the topic but no specific information on the forthcoming lecture. As a result, my knee joints hurt because I wasn't flexible enough to trust that I would receive the information at the appropriate time.

The **skin** reflects how we interface with the world. When the skin is irritated, it is because we perceive the world as abrasive or hostile. If a **boil** develops, that means a specific area of our life is like a sore.

Bones indicate what we inherited from our parents and ancestors, or what we received from genetic memory and early social conditioning.

If an ailment occurs on the **front** of the body, that means we are aware of the issue but we haven't dealt with it yet. If the ailment is on the **back** of the body, we are trying to put it behind us, or we aren't aware of it yet. If it is on the **left** side of the body, it has to do with our feminine aspects, or with female relationships in our life. Problems on the **right** side of the body reflect the masculine part of ourselves, or our masculine relationships.

A **virus** is the result of being invaded—our boundaries have broken down. The first and foremost sacred space for us is our body and we honor ourselves by establishing healthy boundaries and maintaining it.

Viruses, bacteria and fungus invade when our subpersonalities aren't healthy, happy, whole and functioning. Fungus tends to come when we have abandoned ourselves, bacteria invades when deliberate hostile influences are entering our boundaries and viruses are the result of others being allowed to use and abuse us.

Specific body parts

The **head** signals thoughts and ideals—the way we think life ought to be. The **face** has to do with what we are presenting to the world. If our presentation is different from what is actually happening inside, our two "faces" are in conflict. As a result, **acne** may develop.

If we have negative thoughts, resentment, and feelings of being inadequate, mucous will develop in the **sinuses**. Phlegm, the fluid in the **throat**, is also an indication of negative emotions. **Headaches** often constitute repression of memories. They can also signify a conflict between the left and right brains.

For example, our right brain knows that we are all-powerful beings—that every one of us is a consciousness superimposed over All That Is. If the left brain opposes it, we develop a headache.

Ear problems can mean there are things in our environment that we don't wish to hear: abusive language from a spouse; nagging from a mother; or disrespect from a child. When we protect our boundaries, yet realize that we cannot control the behavior of others, this heals. It is also helpful to see the abuse as their reflection, not ours, so that we don't take it personally.

The **thyroid** is where we suppress anger at not being heard. If there are pieces of our reality that don't fit, and we try to ignore them, it effects the thyroid.

Teeth and their roots are connected to bones, therefore, they indicate conflicts with parental figures or societal attitudes. Teeth have to do with how palatable parental teachings were. If we cannot accept a life situation, our teeth may become hypersensitive. Teeth also pertain to the need for aggression.

Problems with **gums** indicate something we cannot swallow in life. It is stuck and bothering us, so it becomes an abscess in the mouth.

The **neck** is where thoughts and ideals meet—reflecting the way life is for us. Light workers often have neck problems because the way they would like life to be and the way life appears, is at variance. That conflict meets in the neck.

A lot of people have **atlas** problems, meaning the head isn't on straight. This indicates a dramatic conflict between ideal and reality and an inability to embrace the folly of mankind. If we can start to see the perfection underlying all things, by looking at the larger picture, this conflict goes away.

The **shoulders, arms** and **hands** reflect that which is done to us or that which we are doing to another. The **hands** indicate the present moment. **Arms** mean it may be less obvious or more under the surface. **Shoulders** indicate that we have been trying to push it into the past.

If our feelings were hurt today, it manifests in the **fingers**. If we are still hurting over something that happened last week, it will possibly manifest in the **arm**, up toward the elbow. If there are issues from our childhood or from past relationships that we suppress, we find that in the **shoulders** or **back**.

Specific areas of the hands indicate different things. The **top joint** or section of the fingers has to do with ideals and the mental. The **middle joint** has to do with emotional issues. The **lower joint** has to do with the physical body. For example, when someone is hostile towards our spiritual beliefs and makes fun of a sacred object or a spiritual book we hold dear, we may develop a problem with the top joint of the finger. If someone makes fun of our intellect or our ability to solve problems, it also manifests in the top joint. One young woman who had developed a huge tumor in the brain came to me. Her husband's favorite nickname for her was "brain dead." That was an insult to the mental and she continually injured the top joints of her fingers.

The area **below the shoulders down to the hips** has to do with our desires and passion and our self-expression of the things we love to do. **Liver** problems indicate anger. **Kidney** problems indicate fear. **Sacrum** problems indicate that we feel unsupported.

The **hip** area is where we balance between how we desire to live and how we are actually living. For example, a man wants to be an artist but his parents forced him to become a lawyer. Therefore, he develops problems in the hips.

The **pubis** bone can lock in the front. There is a cartilage joint that should move, and if it doesn't, it throws the back out of alignment. It locks when our sexuality is being drained. For example, when a young boy is expected to be the man in the family, he may start to shield his masculinity because he feels his energy being drained. If a woman is abused sexually, the pubis will lock.

Sexual organs relate to our ability to be active in reproduction.

Legs reflect how we are moving forward through life. The man who becomes a lawyer instead of an artist may also be prone to hurting his legs. Since his artistic talent is part of his feminine side, and the masculine is crowding it out, it will likely manifest in his left leg.

Knees reflect our flexibility towards what is happening to us. For example, a woman may have a sore right knee when she is being inflexible with her husband.

Problems with the **feet** indicate how we are moving through life in the present moment. For example, a man has many wonderful ideas at his job but his boss won't give him the freedom to follow those ideas, so his masculine side becomes stuck. He may have a car accident and jam the bones of his masculine foot, because his life is jammed from moving forward at this time.

The Body Parts as Dream Symbols

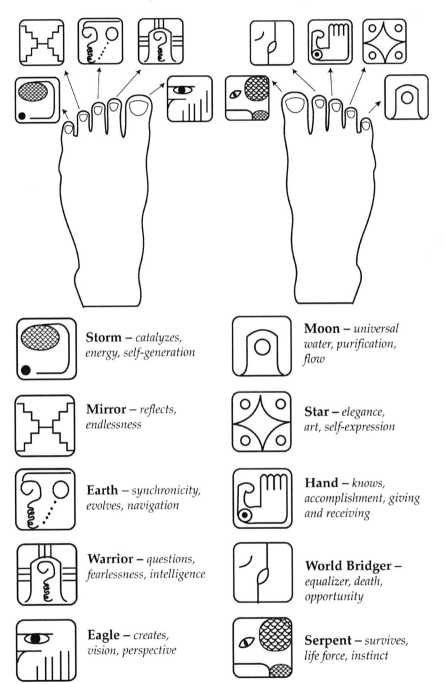

Storm – *catalyzes, energy, self-generation*

Mirror – *reflects, endlessness*

Earth – *synchronicity, evolves, navigation*

Warrior – *questions, fearlessness, intelligence*

Eagle – *creates, vision, perspective*

Moon – *universal water, purification, flow*

Star – *elegance, art, self-expression*

Hand – *knows, accomplishment, giving and receiving*

World Bridger – *equalizer, death, opportunity*

Serpent – *survives, life force, instinct*

The Body Parts as Dream Symbols

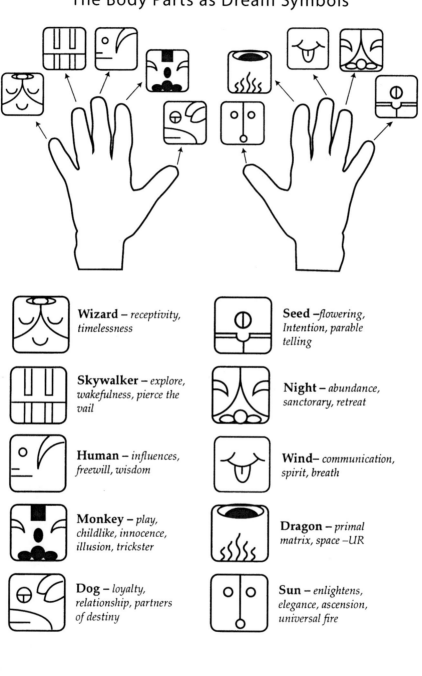

Wizard – *receptivity, timelessness*

Skywalker – *explore, wakefulness, pierce the vail*

Human – *influences, freewill, wisdom*

Monkey – *play, childlike, innocence, illusion, trickster*

Dog – *loyalty, relationship, partners of destiny*

Seed –*flowering, Intention, parable telling*

Night – *abundance, sanctorary, retreat*

Wind– *communication, spirit, breath*

Dragon – *primal matrix, space –UR*

Sun – *enlightens, elegance, ascension, universal fire*

The Body Parts as Dream Symbols

Ankles	flexibility in moving forward in daily life, (left = feminine aspects or relationships of life like spirituality; right = masculine aspects or relationships of life)
Arms	the way others treat you or you treat others (males = right, females = left)
Back	upper—responsibility or ability to carry work load; mid—expression, self-expression; lower—support or lack of
Belly button	sustenance or life force
Blood	love
Bones	parental and hereditary information
Breath	expressing life force
Breasts	nurturing or need of
Chest (lungs)	self-expression when expelling breath, pent-up grief
Colon	letting go of what no longer serves us
Duodenal/transverse colon (solar plexus area)	mothering or insufficient mothering
Ears	desire or ability to hear
Elbows	fluidity in how we treat others
Eyes	desire or ability to see
Feet	ability to move forward
Gall bladder	ability to process density
Genitals	self-perception of one's maleness or female-ness, other—one's maleness/femaleness as reflected by another or, if opposite sex, one's male or female aspects
Hair	social self-image

Hands	relationships
Head	intuition, idealism
Heart	ability to give love
Hips	where the way we want to move through life and the way we move through life meet
Kidneys	fear
Knees	flexibility with relationships and our required roles (left = feminine, right = masculine)
Legs	progress through life
Liver	anger
Mouth	ability to receive sustenance
Neck	ideals vs. reality; the place where the way we want life to be and the way it seems to be, meet
Nose	the right to happiness, to flourish; personal power
Ovaries/testicles	procreation or offspring
Shoulders	responsibility
Skin	interaction with others and outside circumstances
Stomach	acceptance of life's circumstances
Teeth	need for aggression
Thighs	sexuality
Throat	unspoken or spoken words
Wrists	fluidity in relationships

II. INTERPRETING YOUR CHILD'S DREAM IMAGERY

Activities

Acting	authentic expression is needed
Birthing own or other's child	new awareness is about to happen
Biting one's tongue	not the time to speak
Bleeding	leaking resources through loving in a dysfunctional or exploitive way
Boating	need or desire for emotional change
Braiding hair	(self) - integrated self-expression (other) - assisting another in integrating their expression
Breath/breathing	life force; individual expression
Buying	giving power away or exchanging power for approval of others
Can't move	stuck in a world view, or stagnation
Climbing	increasing perception, awareness, consciousness
Cooking	nourishing self and others
Coughing	difficulty to accept
Dancing	self-expression in everyday life, living with grace
Drinking	accepting emotional support (or desire for)
Drowning	feeling suppressed or overpowered
Drunkenness	abandonment of self

Dumping garbage	(others') - they are bringing their unresolved issues into your life (self) - there are old, obsolete issues to be released
Dying	release, fear of success
Eating	self-nourishment
Exercising	preparing for or building energy and power
Falling	fear of failure
Flying	freedom, or need for freedom
Healing injuries	externalizing that which must be
of others	dealt with within
Hunting	self-mastery is needed
Ironing	getting rid of loose ends or minor unresolved issues
Learning in school	humility is needed to learn something
Lessons	pay attention to what is before you, it has something to teach you
Losing hair	losing face or stature in the eyes of others
Losing money	disempowerment
Mending clothes	trying to mend our self-image
Mending roof	holding on to old limitations
Mountain climbing - w/supports - w/attachments to others	life is supporting your hopes others support your hopes
Never-ending work	fear of being overwhelmed or not up to the task

Parachuting	abandoning a world view or life's direction by changing perception
Persecution by authority	fear of victimization
Playing	restoring fun to the journey of life
Playing ball	polarity, seeing opposites, thriving on opposition, causing divisiveness
Purging (vomiting/diarrhea)	releasing unacceptable parts of life
Reading	searching for answers within old world views
Re-injury	recurring karmic issues want to yield their insights
Running	desire for freedom or window of freedom
Running a race	being attached to outcome
Shrinking clothes	hiding behind false humility of others; seeing them as less
Singing	finding your voice or life's calling
Skiing or sledding	our ability to love is too shallow; others can't give us the love we need
Smelling	ability to discern
Smoking (tobacco)	addiction through self-abandonment
Sneezing	desire to express passionately
Spinning	resistance to life, loss of innocence
Stealing	feeling inadequate to provide for ourselves
Suffocating	loss or lack of personal power

Surfing	utilizing an opportunity
Swimming	desire to be loved and accepted
Talking	need to communicate
Teeth falling out	no need for aggression
Teeth being brushed	getting ready for a battle
Theft of money	power has been stolen
Tripping	fear of inadequacy; letting ourselves or others down
Travel	change in or need for awareness (see individual vehicles)
Washing hands	need to put our relationships in order
Winning trophy	need to give self credit; gold for spiritual achievement, silver for worldly achievement
Working	desire or need to take action
Writing	communication
Yawning	need to pull in more energy or resources

Activity, Sexual

This section is recommended for parents of teens and pre-teens

Flirting	desire for vitality
Heterosexual sex	receiving and giving power
Homosexual sex (male)	desire to know one's own maleness; feeling inadequate as a male
Kissing	desire for or lack of energy/power
Lesbian sex	desire to know one's own femaleness; feeling inadequate about being a woman
Masturbation	self-empowerment is needed

Animals

Armadillo	need for defense
Bat	ability or need to find the way through the unknown
Bear	time to go into or come out of seclusion or rest; also rebirth, ending of hardship
Beaver	need to control outcomes, lack of cooperation with one's higher self
Cat	black - black magic white - white magic all others - temporal affairs; everyday activities
Camel	self-reliance, self-sufficiency
Caribou/reindeer	instinct as guidance
Chameleon	fluidity and flexibility needed
Cow	nurturing of others
Crab	warriorship against illusion; spiritual warriorship
Crocodile/alligator	pitfall set up by another
Deer	tranquility and peace
Dinosaur	obsolete supremacies; the old that must be dissolved; obsolete petty tyrants
Dog	relationships, partnerships and friendships
Dolphin	right brain awareness, non-cognitive information, empathic communication
Donkey	allowing others to drain our energy or use us; false humility
Elephant	old patterns or memories
Fox	being tricked into learning the unexpected; expect the unexpected

Frog	experiencing other realms, frequencies or realities; seeing through another's eyes
Hamster	the need to have a spare supply
Hare/rabbit	need for awareness - quick change may be needed; speed is needed
Hippo	need to approach through feeling rather than mind
Horse	balance and freedom in material life
Lion	creation; also destruction
Llama	discovery, sense of adventure
Locust/grasshopper	destruction
Monkey	need to play or playfulness
Mountain goat	leadership, ability to visualize hopes, visionary leadership
Muskox	solidarity, oneness of purpose, well-balanced unity
Octopus	control or confinement of or by another
Penguin	there is far more to something than meets the eye
Platypus	un-integrated, lack of integrity
Raccoon	brashness, impudence; also toughness
Rats/mice	secrets; white rat means hidden insight
Rooster	time to wake up to what's really going on; time to see clearly
Sloth	laziness, lack of self-motivation
Snake	wisdom or need for it
Swan	mastery
Tiger	sovereignty; white tiger means Initiation
Tortoise	the pace is too slow
Turtle	adventurous journey

Vermin	invasion through deceit
Whale	superior wisdom or need for it; creation, creative solutions, new ideas
Wolf	stalking one's own motives or a situation (In Toltec terminology, stalking means to not think we know and to approach with great awareness.)
Wolves howling	need to commune with nature
Wolverine	need to be tough or persevere in the face of greater odds
Worms	decay; something is rotten at the core
Zebra	indecision

Birds

Birds refer to thoughts. Observe the colors (see section on color)

Albatross	detachment from the group; rising above the mundane
Birds of prey	power
Blackbird (except crows)	treachery
Crow/raven	path of power
Dove	peace, tranquility
Eagle	power through perception
Hummingbird	energy; increased resources through timelessness
Owl	seeing or being led thru the dark
Sparrow	fun, joy, being carefree
Turkey	clinging to old patterns or obsolete habits
Vulture	de-structuring; the end of the old

Clothing
Clothing refers to self-image or image to others

Armor	dissolve protectiveness; trust in the benevolence of life
Buttons	unbuttoned – closure is needed buttoned - completion
Coat	need to shield self
Collar	hiding vulnerability
Crown/hat	self importance
Handkerchief	time to get rid of our own or others' negative emotions
Raincoat	resisting the process of life
Shoes	understanding
Socks	that which prevents us from understanding what is really going on behind appearances
Tie	conformity
Underwear	private life
Uniform	assumed authority

Colors

Black	need for wholeness; the unknown
Brown - observe the feeling around it	dirty brown could mean pollution or something unwholesome; clear brown could mean stability or groundedness
Red	need or desire to fight or be aggressive
White	peace/wholeness, purity, high-mindedness
Yellow	spirituality and faith
Green	healing and fertility
Blue	humility and understanding
Pinkish purple	unconditional love

Pink	lightness of being, well-being
Orange	need for shrewdness, cunning, mental strategy
Indigo	need for deeper vision
Violet	mysticism, unseen realms
Turquoise	need to stay centered and go within

Directions

East	direction of sobriety or need to analyze what is behind appearances
West	feeling or need to notice feelings; listening to guidance from inner child
North	place of power and warriorship; viewing the large picture objectively
South	need to meditate or watch dream symbols for guidance, self-nurturing
Right	left-brained, cognitive, masculine aspects of life
Left	intuitive, feminine, spiritual
Above	effortless knowing
Below	instincts should be trusted

Foods

Almond	inter-dimensional communication
Aubergine/eggplant	something appearing very desirable will be less so once experienced
Bread	ability to appreciate and receive daily gifts and blessings
Fish	overcoming appearances; seeing behind face values; something is not what it seems

Grain field	time to reap rewards
Grapes	gifts of life
Grapefruit	bitterness
Honey	delightful results from cooperation
Lemons/limes	sourness
Meat	overcoming old instinctual habits
Milk	easy accomplishments
Nuts in general	worthwhile results once problems are solved
Peas/beans	that which will give more than it takes
Pomegranate	something seeming quite ordinary will reveal greater worth
Potatoes	nurturing the inner life
Pudding	good endings
Pumpkin	that which brings benefits in a fun way
Truffles	buried or suppressed assets

Gems/Jewels/Metals
These refer to great inner gifts

Copper	healing; transmuting harmful energies
Diamond	mastery through overcoming
Emerald	open heart or healing of heart
Garnet	need to trust instincts
Gold	spiritual matters
Pearls	wisdom
Ruby	personal sovereignty, dignity, strength
Sapphire	need for courage and clarity
Silver	everyday matters

Identities/Roles

Angel	protection and guidance from the higher self
Athlete	feeling at home in the body, physical mastery, overcoming the tyranny of the body
Brother	having similar viewpoints or consciousness
Elder	the inner sage personality
Elf	lighthearted playfulness
Engineer	obsolete mental solutions
Giant	beyond expectations
Ghost	something from the past will re-surface if its insights are not gathered or if it is not resolved
Glutton	taking more than is needed
Guest	that which we invite into our life
Guide	listening to inner knowing
Guru	seeking answers outside ourselves
Herald	a new cycle of life has begun
Jester/joker	something is playing a trick on you or making a fool of you
Judge/jury	feeling discriminated against; allowing others to dictate worth or self-worth
Motherhood	self-nurturing of the inner child; self-abandonment through nurturing others;
Military	(navy) - emotional action needed (air force) - mental action needed (army) - action needed in everyday life
Podiatrist	needing advice to understand the next step
Police	when acting protectively, boundaries need to be established; when acting oppressively, victimization or fear thereof

| Priest/preacher | judgmental, obsolete value systems |
| Spouse | being integrated; inner balance or need for it, need for pro-activity and receptivity |

Insects

Insects in general	aspects of shortcomings
Ant	labor or hard work and cooperation needed; drudgery
Bee	cooperation with destiny
Butterfly	spiritual gift; a gift of grace
Hornet/wasp	someone with anger in environment or directed at environment
Moth	gift of power from the cosmos
Spider	shortcomings that feed on ourselves; self-destruction
Termite/louse/ Parasite	allowing others to use us and drain our energy or usurp our life

Miscellaneous

Aristocracy	accessing the inner connection to Source
Christmas	celebrate unity within diversity
December	over-balanced feminine energy; emphasis on emotions
Entrance	receptivity; feed the soul or inner experience
Holiday	back away from what you are doing for a while
Insurance	expecting the worst
January	new resolve, new beginnings
June	over-balance in the masculine or mental

Nature

Air	ability (or lack of) to see behind appearances, to understand what is really going on, mental activity
Caves	subconscious programming
Cliff	trust to make a dramatic change
Clouds	the egoic self; surface mind is obscuring effortless knowing
Darkness	outcomes are undetermined
Desert	despair and hopelessness
Disasters	fear of the future, disempowerment
Earth/soil	groundedness, return to basics, stability
Flower	beauty and grace; dead flower, lack thereof
Forest	shelter and place to rest
Gorse bush	something beautiful or attractive will be injurious or angry
Grass	walking a path with heart and joy
Greenery	fertility, good results in everyday practical matters
Flood	strong flow of emotion
Fog	temporary lack of clarity
Iris	elegance; nobility of character
Jungle	unforeseen adventure
Lava	dramatic changes or de-structuring; destructive release of suppressed need for change
Leaves	(falling) - shed old acquaintances who do not enrich life (on tree) - acquaintances who enrich life
Lightning	dramatic shifts in awareness

Migration of birds	(North) - time for action; time to create new methods and ideas (South) - time for ideas to mature; time to wait, time for beingness
Moon	our dreaming body, intuitive self
Mountain/hill	hope
Ocean	life in general
Open area	need or desire for freedom
Public place	fear of exposure
Rain	the process of life
Rainbow	good will come from seeming disappointment
River	unconditional love
Rock	old memory patterns, old memories
Roots	joy, coming home to oneself
Sand/sea/beach	that which the process of life has taught us
Seed	new beginning that must be nurtured
Shooting star	time to be clear about our wishes
Snow	frozen emotion
Spider web	entrapment or need for freedom from programming
Storm	cataclysmic change
Sun	enlightenment
Sunflower	boldness

Terrain	(muddy) - you can get stuck
	(sand dunes) - slow but comfortable progress
	(sandy) - comfort in your journey
	(snow-topped mountain) - forsaken hopes
	(stony) - way has many abrasive but small obstacles
	(up a cliff) - way is almost impossible
	(up a mountain) - way will be difficult but possible
	(wading through water) - emotions will slow progress; dirty water, unpleasant emotions
	(with boulders) - big obstacles are ahead
Valley	place of security
Waves of the ocean	opportunities
Wind	thought that will change perspectives

Numbers

0	completion
1	interconnectedness of life, oneness
2	humility and understanding needed
3	trust the intuitive
4	stability and balance or need for
5	freedom and change
6	guidance within physical life
7	enlightenment
8	opening or closing of a cycle; harmonious interaction
9	feminine side of spiritual gifts; alchemy, intuition, non-cognitive information

10	inclusiveness, not thinking in a separative way
11	transformation or need for; chance to go to the next level
12	strength and power, enlightenment
13	new birth or beginnings

Objects

Ashes	remnants of the old
Ball	if it's your turn to throw it, action is required; if you're catching it you have just received a challenge
Balloon	not having much substance
Bandage	not dealing with the root of the issue; a cover up
Basement	sub-conscious, hidden flaws
Basket	cooperative support, unity within diversity
Beads	parts of a greater achievement; cooperative accomplishment
Bell	praiseworthy emotions waiting to be expressed
Bible	over-inflated value through conditioned programming
Blanket	comfort through denial
Books	looking for answers within the prison bars of social learning
Boxes	something hidden in a box means secrets kept; storage boxes mean that which we have put behind us; boxes in general are limitations through social conditioning
Branch	disconnection from Source

Bricks/building	one step at a time; a belief system blocks is forming to trap your awareness
Bridge	time for a change in lifestyle
Brush	(see comb)
Buildings	view of the world, perspective through social conditioning
Cage	loss of freedom
Candle/lamp	guidance through perception; guidance from unseen realms
Ceiling	limitation
Chimney	outlet for anger
Church	seeking peace and contentment without
City/town/village	common world view or social conditioning
Claw	open attack, greed or aggression
Clock	(alarm) time to wake up; indicates time for change; when we're late it means change or action is overdue
Comb	a few unresolved issues waiting to give their insights
Crayon	spontaneous expression
Crown	arrogant self-opinion
Cross/crucifix	caution; others will turn against or falsely accuse you
Comet	self-achievement; authentic self-expression
Cupboards/closets	the subconscious; events that have not yielded their insights
Curtains	fear of exposure or that which obscures vision
Dam/lake	conditional or conditioned love
Dart	need to protect yourself, become less of a target

Desk	immediate decisions need to be made
Doll	substitution of the artificial for the real
Door	possibilities
Dripping tap	suppressed emotions leaking into life
Eggs	fertility awaiting birth
Egg yolks	the luminous cocoon of man
Engine	the tyranny of social pressure
Excavation	find resources or perception deep inside
Factory	joyless labor, heartless drudgery; need to combine work and joy
Farm	independence, self-reliance
Feces	money or desire for money
Fire	de-structuring or dramatic change
Flag	a cause; patriotism
Flagpole	without a cause, devoid of motive
Floor	perspective of life, world-view
Food	spiritual nurturing
Furniture	(bed) - need or desire to rest (chair) - comfort zone (lamp) - illumination or guidance (screen) - something obscuring vision (table) - decisive action needed
Gallows	others will judge you or you are condemning another
Garbage	that which needs to be discarded
Gift or gift wrap	there are unseen gifts and benefits
Glasses - sun glasses	the need to see clearly pessimism; negativity
Gloves	if removed, need for directness or 'tough love'; if put on, something must be treated delicately

Goggles	see the root cause of strong emotion
Glue	something will be hard to get rid of
Gymnasium	push beyond present boundaries, beyond mortal boundaries
Handbag	potential power
Harp	the need to soothe or be soothed
Hearing	ability to receive guidance
Hotel	belief systems received from others
Inkspot	blemish in purity
Key	solution or missing piece; missing puzzle piece indicates the same
Kite	getting an idea or project off the ground
Laboratory	alchemy, combination of parts for a greater whole
Ladder	ascending consciousness
Lamp post	you are cosmically guided
Law	the tyranny of an obsolete system
Lawn	conformity; conformity of expression
Lighthouse/foghorn	watch for a sign about avoiding certain things in your life
Lock w/o a key	not accessible at this time
Lock of hair	sentimental programs
Locket	a cherished memory is binding you to that which no longer serves
Luggage	encumbered by past burdens
Magnifying glass	details have been overlooked
Manure	feeding on the obsolete, looking to the old for spiritual nourishment
Metronome	something dictating the pace of life

Monastery	need to bring living space into harmony with the inner world; need to disconnect from a life of illusion and materialism
Money	crystallized power
Monument	value systems; socially conditioned values
Music	harmonious interaction
Musical instruments	(percussion) - harmony with destiny (string) - harmony within relationships (wind) - harmony with concepts/thoughts
Musical notes	past life issues or memories
Newspaper	common view of the world
Palace	complexity created by mind
Pennies	undervalued power and ability
Pets	companionship
Photos	events or interactions that have not yet yielded their insights; events that need closure
Playpen	spontaneity is being suppressed
Pots & pans	tools of spiritual nourishment
Prism	seeing with separation consciousness
Prison	the need to let go of belief systems
Racquet	'the ball is in your court', it is time to act
Record (musical)	get out of the rut
Religious artifacts	self-righteousness, belief systems of status and self-importance
Report card (grades)	time to account for ourselves; time to live what we know
Reward	(money) a gift of power (trophy) acknowledgement

Ribbons	pink means innocence; white means according to divine will; red means do not proceed; black means death
Riddles	do not try to understand; that which is real is indefinable
Ring	inclusiveness; power through aligning with Infinite will
Road sign	an advisable course of action on your life's journey
Rocket	rapid accomplishment
Roof	self-imposed limitation
Rust	that which is no longer life-enhancing
Secret mission or agent	destiny
School	the need to learn
Sight	ability to see behind appearances
Smoke	indication of suppressed anger
Soap	clean up an area of your life
Spear	protect against the vindictiveness of another
Spiral	finding inner silence
Stairs	going up or down in levels of awareness
Stage play	lack of authenticity
Tablecloth	tactful action needed
Target	goal is in sight or focus
Taste	nurturing, self-nurturing or spiritual nurturing
Telephone	inter-dimensional communication wishes to express; listen in silent meditation
Telescope	deepen your perception

Toilet	obsolete needs to be released; if over-flowing, getting rid of the old is overdue
Tools	assets and talents - Ex.: a broom might mean you need to clean up a portion of your life. A certain quality or the need for that quality.
Tracks	residue, remaining influence
Treadmill	stuck in a no-win situation
Treasure	multiple gifts, opportunities or abilities will be given at once
Umbrella	clinging to old viewpoints and belief systems, holding on to old limitations
Video/movie	surface appearances are not real
Walls	blockage of perception, being trapped by labels or belief systems
Washing machine	cleansing old ways of relating to others, cleansing old self-images
Water - flooding the floor	emotion emotions sweeping away old foundational beliefs
Well	deep, un-surfaced emotion
Wings	passion, exploration
Wool on a sheep	insulate your sacred space
Wound	unprocessed pain that has not yielded its insights; pain that has not been valued
Wreck of a vehicle	the old way of moving through life must immediately be changed
Weapons	need to protect yourself
Wheels	primary supporting relationships
Window	vision, ideals

Zipper	unzipped = exclusiveness, separateness zipped = inclusiveness

Transportation

Air	changes in perception, ideas or ideals
Animal	change in aspect represented by animal; i.e., donkey = false humility
Bicycle	seeing opposites as having unequal value; duality
Car	the way we travel thru life, e.g., jobs, relationships
Going backwards	slipping back into old habits
Hearse/funeral procession	something must be eliminated for aware- ness to progress
Public (bus/train)	change in social conditioning
Road	change in general awareness, direction
Skates	adventurous fun
Skis	hopeful anticipation
Sled/sleigh	superficial, shallow living

OTHER BOOKS BY ALMINE

Almine is the author of 10 books, a number of which have been translated into several languages. Other books she has written that are recommended for parental guidance are:

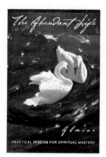

The Abundant Life
By popular demand, the profound words of wisdom that have changed the lives of more than 20,000 daily Twitter followers, communicating in multiple languages, have been compiled into book form.

Three hundred aphorisms and mandalas from the Seer Almine will delight and inspire her growing global audience.

Published: 2010, 188 pages, soft cover, 6 x 9, $19.95
ISBN: 978-1-934070-20-8

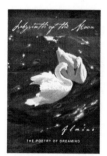

Labyrinth of the Moon
The book contains 144 verses of the Poetry of Dreaming and extensive lists of the interpretations of dream symbols. It is a valuable tool for opening up the deeper dream-state's communications, promoting the healing of the psyche, the body and facilitating the balance of the Inner Child and other sub-personalities.

Designed to release the hold of past incarnational cycles, it is an essential companion for practitioners of Shrihat Satva Yoga.

Published: 2010, 250 pages, soft cover, 6 x 9, $19.95
ISBN: 978-1-934070-10-9

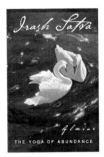

Irash Satva Yoga

The human body is unique in that it is an exact microcosm of the macrocosm of created life. There are 12 points along the right, masculine side of the body and the same number on the left side. These are microcosmic replicas of the macrocosmic cycles of life.

The yoga postures are designed to open and remove the debris from these points – the gates of dreaming. This will occur physically through the postures and the music. Dissolving debris also occurs by way of dreaming (triggered by the breathing and eye movements), releasing past issues that caused the blockages in the points.

Published: 2010, 112 pages, soft cover, 6 x 9, $24.95
ISBN: 978-1-934070-95-6

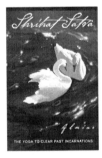

Shrihat Satva Yoga

The human body is unique in that it is an exact microcosm of the macrocosm of created life. There are 12 points along the right, masculine side of the body and the same number on the left side. These are microcosmic replicas of the macrocosmic cycles of life.

The yoga postures are designed to open and remove the debris from these points – the gates of dreaming. This will occur physically through the postures and the music. Dissolving debris also occurs by way of dreaming (triggered by the breathing and eye movements), releasing past issues that caused the blockages in the points.

Published: 2010, 80 pages, soft cover, 6 x 9, $34.95
ISBN: 978-1-934070-15-4

To order, call toll-free: 877 552-5646
or order online:
http://www.spiritualjourneys.com